KV-457-500

Standard Haematology Practice

Dr. P. A. E. Jones
Consultant Haematologist
Department Of Haematology
City Hospital
Nottingham NG5 1PB

Telephone 0602 627708

Standard Haematology Practice

Edited by Bryon Roberts
on behalf of the British Committee
for Standards in Haematology

Foreword by A.H. Waters
Chairman, British Committee for Standards in Haematology

OXFORD
BLACKWELL SCIENTIFIC PUBLICATIONS
LONDON EDINBURGH BOSTON
MELBOURNE PARIS BERLIN VIENNA

© 1991 by
Blackwell Scientific Publications
Editorial Offices:
Osney Mead, Oxford OX2 0EL
25 John Street, London WC1N 2BL
23 Ainslie Place, Edinburgh EH3 6AJ
3 Cambridge Center, Cambridge
Massachusetts 02142, USA
54 University Street, Carlton
Victoria 3053, Australia

Other Editorial Offices:
Arnette SA
2, rue Casimir-Delavigne
75006 Paris
France

Blackwell Wissenschaft
Meinekestrasse 4
D-1000 Berlin 15
Germany

Blackwell MZV
Feldgasse 13
A-1238 Wien
Austria

All rights reserved. No part of this publication may be reproduced, stored in a retrieval system, or transmitted, in any form or by any means, electronic, mechanical, photocopying, recording or otherwise without the prior permission of the copyright owner.

First published 1991

Set by Times Graphics, Singapore
Printed and bound in Great Britain by
Hartnolls Ltd, Bodmin, Cornwall

DISTRIBUTORS

Marston Book Services Ltd
PO Box 87
Oxford OX2 0DT
(*Orders*: Tel: 0865 791155
Fax: 0865 791927
Telex: 837515)

USA
Mosby–Year Book, Inc.
11830 Westline Industrial Drive
St Louis, Missouri 63146
(*Orders*: Tel: 800 633-6699)

Canada
Mosby–Year Book, Inc.
5240 Finch Avenue East
Scarborough, Ontario
(*Orders*: Tel: 416 298-1588)

Australia
Blackwell Scientific Publications
(Australia) Pty Ltd
54 University Street
Carlton, Victoria 3053
(*Orders*: Tel: 03 347-0300)

British Library
Cataloguing in Publication Data

Standard haematology practice
1. Medicine. Diagnosis. Haematology
I. Roberts, Bryon
616. 07561

ISBN 0-632-02623-5

Contents

List of Contributors

General Haematology Task Force

J.M. England (*Chairman*); R.M. Rowan (*Secretary*); M. Brozović; D.W. Dawson; S.M. Lewis; N.K. Shinton; A.D. Stephens; D.P. Thomas.

Past Members and Contributors
A.J. Bellingham; A.J. Birch; A.N. Lestas; L. Luzzato; the late G.W. Marsh.

Haemostasis and Thrombosis Task Force

J.F. Davidson (*Chairman*); B.T. Colvin (*Secretary*); T.W. Barrowcliffe; P.B.A. Kernoff; S.J. Machin; F.E. Preston; I.D. Walker.

Past Members and Contributors
The late P. Barkhan; D.W. Dawson; E.E. Mayne; R.S. Mibashan; L. Poller; N.K. Shinton; D.P. Thomas, J.M. Thomson.

Blood Transfusion Task Force

D. Voak (*Chairman*); J.A.F. Napier (*Secretary*); F.E. Boulton; R. Cann; R.D. Finney; I.D. Fraser; A.N. Horn; W. Wagstaff; A.H. Waters; J.K. Wood.

Past Members and Contributors
J.F. Davidson; D.W. Dawson; K.M. Forman; H.H. Gunson; R.C. Knight; E.E. Lloyd; G.D. Poole; A.J. Rejman; A. Smithies; M. Scott.

Clinical Haematology Task Force

J.A. Whittaker (*Chairman*); D. Gorst (*Secretary*); N.C. Allan; A.J. Bellingham; V. Clough; I.M. Franklin; A.J. Rejman; G. Smith.

Past Members and Contributors
I.W. Delamore; I.D. Fraser; P. Mosley; E.A.E. Robinson.

British Committee for Standards in Haematology

A.H. Waters (*Chairman*); J.K. Wood (*Secretary*); T.W. Barrowcliffe; M. Brozović; J.F. Davidson; M. Fuller; J.C. Giddings; A.V. Hoffbrand; W. Muir; A.J. Rejman; R.M. Rowan; N.H. Russell; D. Voak; J.A. Whittaker.

Foreword

The British Committee for Standards in Haematology (BCSH) is a standing sub-committee of the British Society for Haematology (BSH). It was founded in 1964 in response to an invitation from the newly formed International Committee for Standards in Haematology (ICSH) and sends a representative to the assembly of that Committee.

The aims and composition of the BCSH have evolved since then. Its objective is to maintain standards in all branches of haematology throughout the United Kingdom linked with parallel work at an international level. The BCSH works closely with the External Quality Assessment Schemes in Haematology, Blood Coagulation and Blood Group Serology to investigate problem areas in laboratory practice and, where appropriate, to organize educational workshops.

The composition of the Committee was changed in 1987 to include representatives from those societies and organizations, in addition to the BSH, who have a major interest in the objectives of the BCSH. These currently include the British Blood Transfusion Society, the British Society for Haemostasis and Thrombosis and the Institute of Medical Laboratory Sciences.

The BCSH is advised by its expert Task Forces in General Haematology, Clinical Haematology, Blood Transfusion and Haemostasis and Thrombosis. The Committee and its Task Forces have had a very prolific period since 1984 as the reader will see from the many guidelines on various aspects of haematology and blood transfusion practice which are included in this compendium. It has been a privilege to be associated with the BCSH during this period, and latterly as its Chairman.

Professor A.H. Waters
St Bartholomew's Hospital and
Medical College, London

Editor's Comments

Guidelines on various topics have been produced by the British Committee for Standards in Haematology (BCSH) on behalf of the British Society for Haematology (BSH) for some years now. This book collects together those that have been produced by the Task Forces of the BCSH since 1984.

All the guidelines have been recently reviewed and apart from those on Computing in General Haematology, Computing in Hospital Blood Banks, Heparin Therapy and Haemoglobinopathy Screening, have been virtually rewritten. In fact Chapters 1, 2, 3 and 4 are new and as yet unpublished guidelines. Each chapter represents the considerable efforts of a working party or Task Force together with further constructive modification by the main Committee (BCSH) before being finally approved by the BSH Committee. The chapters on blood transfusion were prepared jointly with members of the British Blood Transfusion Society. Chapter 18 was based on a report of a working party of the Regional Transfusion Directors of the National Blood Transfusion Service and the assistance of the Royal College of Nursing is also recognized in the preparation of Chapter 19.

My task as editor has been the relatively easy one of collating the results of the hard labours of others. The names of the members of the various Task Forces and their working parties are given. Every effort has been made not to omit any names but with recent revisions and changes in membership of committees this task has been made difficult. My apologies are presented in full, however, should any name be missing. This book represents a massive effort by many experts in British haematology and my thanks are to them all.

B.E. Roberts

Disclaimer

Whilst the (advice and) information contained in this book is believed to be true and accurate at the date of going to press, neither the author nor the publisher can accept any legal responsibility or liability for any errors or omissions that may be made.

1 Code for Good Laboratory Practice in Haematology Laboratories (Including Hospital Blood Banks)

Prepared by the
General Haematology Task Force*

Introduction

Modern laboratory practice requires planning and managerial skills as well as the technical competence and scientific innovation which have been the hallmark of the diagnostic service unit. The work of the laboratory must be justified in terms of the applicability and practical relevance of the procedures which are carried out, ability to function within defined cost limits and an assurance that the laboratory is a safe place in which to work.

This chapter is intended to provide guidance for the application of a code of practice in the haematology laboratory, so as to establish a consistently high standard of performance in achieving these objectives. The haematology laboratory should provide investigative services and therapeutic products for haemostasis and thrombosis and hospital blood banking, in addition to general haematology services.

Definitions

Planning is defined as the methodical and logical selection of a series of complementary actions for the purpose of pursuing and achieving an objective.

Management is the process of planning; organizing; training; motivating and controlling staff; and developing procedures to achieve defined goals.

Operation is the sum of the different activities in any enterprise.

Budgeting is the maintenance of the financial equilibrium of the enterprise.

Responsibilities

These are separated into two components, administrative and operational.

* With contributions from D. Voak (Chair of Blood Transfusion Task Force) and J.F. Davidson (Chair of Haemostasis Task Force).

Administrative responsibility

Administrative responsibility includes the following factors.

JOB SPECIFICATIONS

A job specification defines those requirements, both professional and personal, which best suit an individual for a given job.

TERMS AND CONDITIONS OF SERVICE

A job description defines those tasks which an individual in employment is expected to perform and serves to protect the employee. In addition, it should describe conditions of service, for example salary, hours of work, annual leave, etc.

SCHEDULING OF WORK

Personnel must be available when work requires to be done, but since staff account for the largest cost in any operation, strenuous efforts must be made to ensure their most effective utilization. Particular attention must be paid to any requirement for emergency duties. Adequate staff, both medical and technical, at appropriate levels of skill, are required.

SELECTION OF INVESTIGATIONS AND PROCEDURES

Choice will be determined by: clinical requirements; number of requests; practical complexity of the procedure; margins of error which are tolerable; degree of urgency for results; ability to interpret results; availability of appropriately trained staff; availability of equipment and ease of preventive maintenance of equipment; the availability, shelf-life and cost of reagents; ability to 'trouble-shoot'; purchase and running costs; and finally safety considerations.

DESCRIPTION OF PROCEDURES

The preparation of procedure manuals is a prime responsibility of the consultant haematologist in charge in collaboration with appropriate individuals. This should include not only detailed method descriptions but standard procedures for all laboratory operations. These include patient preparation, sample handling, preventive maintenance, quality control, all record systems, communication of results and comments, inventory and safety procedures for the protection of staff in the event of accidents involving chemical agents, physical agents and risk of infection. Finally all laboratories should define, in detail, the procedures to be followed in the event of a major accident. Good laboratory practice dictates that operating procedures should be in writing and should be regularly reviewed. These documents should be made available to all employees. Management should ensure that they have been read and understood.

DEFINITION OF QUALITY ASSURANCE PROCEDURES*

This must include all aspects of both non-analytical and analytical quality assurance.

SAFETY OF STAFF

This requires the creation of an environment in which laboratory workers can and are trained to operate without hazard or alternatively where hazards are identified and unambiguous procedures for treatment are clearly displayed in the event of accidents arising from these hazards. Where necessary, national guidelines should be consulted, for example concerning hepatitis and HIV infection. A safety officer must be appointed.

FINANCIAL CONTROL

See section on Purchasing Policy and Maintenance Contracts, p. 14.

STATUTORY REGULATIONS AND LEGAL RESPONSIBILITIES

Management staff must be aware of relevant statutory regulations (Health and Safety Commission, 1975) including product liability (Department of Trade and Industry, 1987; DHSS, 1988) in addition to legal responsibilities. Ignorance of these is never an acceptable plea in mitigation in a court of law. In addition, it is necessary to ensure that all staff are informed of such regulations and responsibilities where relevant. Administrative responsibility can only be held by an individual who by virtue of training and experience can reasonably be expected to perform these duties to an adequate standard.

STAFF–MANAGEMENT CONSULTATION

A procedure should be established which permits consultation between senior laboratory management and trade union representatives.

* As defined by ICSH (1986): see Appendix.

STAFF TRAINING AND EDUCATION

This may be provided 'in service' by educational establishments, professional organizations, government agencies or by manufacturers. Library facilities should be available.

Operational responsibility

Operational responsibility includes the following:

1 distribution of duties
2 supervision of work
3 supervision of quality assurance
4 supervision of reporting and records
5 compliance with operating procedures
6 compliance with statutory regulations and legal responsibilities
7 maintenance of equipment and updating of procedures.

Facilities

Minimum criteria for facilities must be defined for each laboratory. Failure to attain these minimum criteria precludes the adequate and safe performance of procedures. In general, facilities must be sufficient to permit the performance of a test with defined precision and accuracy and without endangering the operator or any third party. Included under this heading are:

1 space (laboratory and administrative functions, storage)
2 services (special requirements for equipment, environment, telephone)
3 furnishings
4 equipment
5 materials
6 staff facilities
7 information technology.

It is important to appreciate that laboratory instrumentation may require additional facilities such as air conditioning, special electrical outlets and extra plumbing.

Standard operating procedures

Comprehensive unambiguous written operating procedures should be available covering all aspects of laboratory practice. Procedures should be described in a step-by-step format and include details of patient preparation, specimen collection and handling, test materials, test procedures, calibration procedures, quality control, interpretation of test results, safety precautions and references. It is useful to preface the procedure method by a brief description of the principle of the test and the main clinical indications for its use. The following procedures should be described.

Patient reception, preparation and sample handling

Technical methods

Description of technical methods should include not only step-by-step detail of technique and its quality control but also procedures for preventive maintenance and simple 'trouble-shooting'. Similar written procedures should be available for use of diagnostic reagents, including kits.

Data flow and communication

In addition to the issue of reports the laboratory must keep a complete set of recorded results which are immediately available. It is important to appreciate that just like the patient's case record, laboratory results are confidential and adequate arrangements must be made to assure their confidentiality. At the same time, however, clear lines for communicating results from laboratory to clinician must be defined. Appropriate 'reference intervals' must be used, obtained from healthy reference sample groups and possibly other interesting reference sample groups with well specified disorders (ICSH 1981). Critical values demanding immediate clinical attention must be defined and clearly communicated to laboratory personnel.

Quality assurance

This is a programme for assuring reliability of results and must be viewed in totality by including all components of non-analytical quality assurance as well as the better recognized processes of internal analytical quality control* and external quality assessment.* A Quality Assurance Officer should be appointed from amongst the staff of the department(s) to ensure the introduction of and adherence to the programme. This individual will be directly responsible to the head of the department and will ensure the application of quality assurance by acting in conjunction with the most senior Medical Laboratory Scientific Officer (MLSO) in each section of the laboratory.

* As defined by ICSH (1986): see Appendix.

NON-ANALYTICAL QUALITY ASSURANCE

Quality assurance includes ensuring that specimens are collected correctly, are adequately anticoagulated if so required, are transported to the laboratory without delay, and are maintained at appropriate ambient temperature before analysis. It continues within the laboratory (see below) and also includes ensuring that reports are not delayed after completion of tests.

Proper procedures must be established for receipt of specimens in the laboratory. These must be transported in separate plastic bags; request forms must be placed in a separate pocket of the bag to avoid contamination but arranged so as not to be separated from the specimen until well matched in the laboratory. On arrival in the laboratory, specimens must be checked for correct type of container, for the correct amount of blood in relation to anticoagulant and for the condition of the specimen. Leaking specimens must be discarded (see below). Unreasonable delays between collection of specimens and receipt in laboratory must be investigated.

Request forms and specimen containers must have adequate identification; if any specimen is labelled inadequately to ensure correct identification, that specimen should not be analysed. Specimens should be given a laboratory number and details should be entered into a current paper file or computer by an MLSO or by clerical staff who will at this stage identify potentially hazardous specimens in accordance with a list of 'high risk' conditions or by the presence of a warning label on the specimens and/or request forms. Such specimens and any leaking specimens (see above) will be brought to the attention of senior technical or a medical member of the laboratory staff and will require special handling. Similarly, urgent specimens should be identified and dealt with separately to ensure rapid analysis.

The head of the laboratory will establish the practice of the laboratory with regard to preparing blood films, and where relevant the criteria for either manual/visual differential leucocyte counts or screening by automated counter.

While blood counts and other tests are generally analysed by MLSOs, the head will establish the policy for examination of stained blood films by MLSOs and medical staff. Bone marrow films and biopsies will be examined and reported by medical staff.

Detailed instructions should be given for the correct transcription of results to report forms or to computer-generated result sheets. Staff performing the work should ensure that the results are technically valid and that an appropriate quality control programme has been used. All reports should be scrutinized and validated by senior MLSOs in accordance with a protocol which has been laid down by the head. Urgent results should be scrutinized by a senior MLSO and reported as 'provisional'. If a report has been telephoned, this should be noted in the laboratory record. The consultant haematologist, head of department, will also establish procedures for the investigation of haemostatic disorders and the control of anticoagulant therapy. The head of department will establish a policy for the interpretation, further investigation if required and communication of the results to the requesting clinician along with advice on blood product therapy, as appropriate, by medical staff.

ANALYTICAL QUALITY CONTROL

For good laboratory practice it is mandatory to have an established set of procedures for internal quality control and to participate in the National External Quality Assessment Schemes. In the general haematology NEQAS each Consultant Haematologist, head of laboratory, elects to nominate an individual contact who receives the survey samples and the subsequent reports and performance analyses. The head is ultimately responsible for the laboratory performance and should review results with the named contact regularly. Conversely, when the head is the contact he or she must review the results with the most senior MLSO and the quality assurance officer.

The internal quality control programme should be realistic, but every procedure and all reagents should be evaluated according to a practical schedule. For qualitative and semi-quantitative tests the frequency of this should be in direct proportion to the frequency with which faults are discovered. For quantitative tests control material* should be included at regular intervals. A record must be maintained of all results of quality control procedures including those for analyses which were not reported because of technical failures as well as results of check tests on reagents, stains and kits.

The total procedure for each laboratory will vary with the circumstances, but at least some of the following programme must be carried out.

1 At appropriate intervals, for example not less than twice each day for blood cell counters, control material must be included as samples in the analytical procedure. Results for patient samples should not be issued until it is clear that no change in the process has occurred. Once this has been demonstrated results may be issued with confidence.

Control materials may be prepared in the laboratory or obtained commercially. During their preparation they must undergo testing in accordance with established health and safety practice. When human blood is used it should, as far as possible, be prepared from donations which have been tested individually for HIV antibody and for hepatitis B surface antigen, and shown to be negative. When it is necessary to use untested blood, this fact should be indicated on the label and the sample should be regarded as potentially infectious and treated

* As defined by ICSH (1986): see Appendix.

with the same precautions as patients' specimens. The essential requirements for using control materials are: (i) sterility; (ii) stability for an identifiable period during which it can be used; (iii) representative distribution from stock; (iv) comparability to blood in behaviour in the test procedure, at least within identified limits; and (v) for quantitative tests mean and Standard Deviation (SD) values established on the batch by replicate tests (at least 10 measurements) under standardized conditions. Some commercial control materials are supplied with assigned values. Only material which is designated as a calibrator* and which has a stated value that has been determined by a reference method* should be used for instrument calibration.

2 In laboratories with computer facilities, when the population of patients from whom the laboratory's samples are drawn remains stable, it may be possible to use the estimate of the total daily or weekly patient mean of absolute values (MCV, MCH, MCHC) for monitoring the occurrence of drift. However, before patient data are used, it is essential to establish the stability of the patient population from day-to-day and within any sub-batches that may be analysed. Laboratories which cannot demonstrate the stability of the sample populations must not use patients' data to monitor their activities.

3 As a further check of precision,* duplicate measurements should be performed on specimens in a test batch taken randomly from the batch.

4 Correlation of results of related investigations, for example blood count and blood film appearances, provides a means of checking on the test performance. The use of cumulative report forms for each patient is a useful way to demonstrate a changed value from one day to the next. When a change occurs which does not correspond to a recognizable cause it is essential to check that this has not been due to an incorrectly identified sample or other clerical error.

Hospital blood banking

The primary objective of the hospital blood bank is to ensure the safe and efficient provision of compatible blood for transfusion. This is achieved by a series of quality assurance procedures enabling validation of each step in the overall process. Many of these steps are entirely within laboratory control. Others, however, are external activities and include collection of blood specimens at the bedside and the administration of blood units. Despite this, their performance must meet the stringent requirements set by the laboratory (see Chapter 12). The security of the entire operation is determined by the weakest link in the organizational chain.

Blood bank computers combined with automated blood grouping machines improve the standard of blood typing by reducing both clerical errors and

* As defined by ICSH (1986): see Appendix.

technical variations. Although blood bank computers are in use in many laboratories, the workload of the laboratory may not justify the cost of an automated blood typing machine. Most hospital blood banks still rely on manual techniques. Blood group serology must be evaluated by control procedures which will demonstrate satisfactory performance of both reagents and techniques (see Chapter 14). The requirement for a stringent approach has been clearly demonstrated by the high incidence of false negative errors in compatibility tests judged by external proficiency trials (Holburn, 1982).

The hospital blood bank should define a series of quality control procedures which will ensure safe and accurate transfusion practice. There must be established, and defined in Standing Operating Procedures, an 'in-house' approach for the identification, prevention and correction of errors.

QUALITY ASSURANCE IN BLOOD BANKING

Safe transfusion practice can be achieved by focusing quality assurance through a correctly organized scheme of management. This requires clearly identified individual levels of responsibility, properly trained personnel and laboratories which have been adequately designed and equipped (AABB, 1981). The major areas requiring attention in a quality control programme are:

1 documentation of blood specimens and patient identity
2 standard operating procedures for all procedures, technical and clerical, within the laboratory
3 specification and quality control of
  (a) reagents (Voak & Napier, 1989)
  (b) techniques (Chapter 14)
  (c) equipment
Analytical quality assurance by external proficiency and in-house exercises
4 transportation and storage of specimens and blood/blood products
5 arrangements for the administration of blood units at the bedside
6 development of a reliable reporting system for errors and adverse reactions
7 continuous education programme to stimulate interest and development programme to improve techniques and efficiency.

DOCUMENTATION AND CLERICAL PROCEDURES

Safety in hospital blood banking depends on accurate patient and specimen identification at all stages in the procedure, commencing with collection of the blood specimen from the patient for compatibility testing and ending with the transfusion of the blood. Clerical procedures in the laboratory must follow a standard procedure (see Chapters 12 and 13). The request form for blood and blood products must give the full name, case record number, date of birth, address and relevant clinical history. Errors of identity can only be avoided if double checks of request form and specimen are carried out at the bedside by the person obtaining the venous specimen and in the laboratory by the person performing the compatibility test.

STANDARD OPERATING PROCEDURES (SOP)

To maintain consistency, safety and security of performance, all laboratory activities must be performed in accordance with clearly written instructions, authorized by the consultant haematologist who is head of department. These require regular review and the date of any revision clearly recorded. Obsolete SOPs must be removed from circulation. SOPs should include the following:

1 title of procedure and brief description of its purpose

2 description of the scientific principles supported by references where necessary

3 specifications for reagents and equipment

4 details of method and an example of work protocol

5 quality control procedures

6 specification for personnel and training requirements

7 detail of health and safety requirements.

SPECIFICATION AND QUALITY CONTROL OF REAGENTS—GENERAL PRINCIPLES

Only reagents made to high specifications should be selected. There should be a remaining shelf-life of 6 months at the time of purchase where possible. National reference preparations are being established for ABO and Rh D reagents. Colour dyes if used in reagents should follow the code established by the US Food and Drug Administration (Hoppe, 1979) of blue for anti-A, yellow for anti-B and green for AHG. Reagents should be used according to the manufacturer's instructions and must be restandardized if they are to be used by alternative techniques or in a diluted form. Any new reagent must be compared against the current reagent to ensure reliability. Parallel testing over 30–50 blood specimens is required to ensure that the new reagent is at least as good as the previous one. Routine quality control of antibody reagents should be based on the use of both positive and negative controls with each batch of tests to demonstrate that the reagents are both specific and potent.

Agglutination reactions should be graded and recorded in a standardized manner. The following is recommended by Voak and Napier (1989):

Symbol	*Agglutinates*
C	One clump
+ + +	Several clumps
+ +	Smaller clumps
+	Granules
(+)	Small granules
W	Microscopic agglutination only
–	Negative

The saline or phosphate buffered saline used for titration studies should always contain 1–3% bovine albumin to prevent adhesion of agglutinates to the surface of glass tubes. Human serum-derived reagents can only be used if the individual donations used to prepare the product have been tested and found negative for HIV antibody and HBsAg. This must be clearly stated on the container. However, no test method can offer complete assurance that products derived from human blood will not transmit infection. They must therefore be handled with extreme caution.

ROUTINE QUALITY CONTROL OF EQUIPMENT

Like reagents, the performance of laboratory equipment must not be assumed. Measurements should be monitored on a regular basis and the results recorded. Cleanliness of equipment must be maintained on a regular basis for the safety of both patients and staff. A programme incorporating the following procedures should be adopted:

1 monitoring of the performance of blood storage refrigerators, laboratory refrigerators, freezers, incubators and water-baths at each time of use. A permanent continuous record of blood storage refrigerators should be made

2 automatic washers for Anti Human Globulin (AHG) tests should be checked by replicate tests twice each week

3 centrifuges should be checked weekly to ensure freedom from faults and that their calibration has not altered (blood bag centrifuges in particular should be checked for accuracy of speed and time controls every 2 months)

4 pH meters should be checked by means of control solutions on each occasion that they are used

5 a preventive maintenance schedule should be established in conjunction with appropriate engineering or electrical staff or contracted outside specialists.

Maintenance of equipment

New equipment should undergo a limited evaluation* on installation, prior to being put into service. Thereafter, a schedule for regular inspection and

* As defined by ICSH (1984).

maintenance must be drawn up and rigorously followed. The schedule should be based on the manufacturer's recommendations and on good practice (Table 1.1).

Inventory management

The procurement of laboratory supplies is greatly facilitated by an inventory system which identifies all supply needs and the quantity of items to be kept immediately available. The system must allow personnel both a means of

Table 1.1 Good practice for maintenance of equipment

Type of apparatus	Type of maintenance	Frequency
Cell counter*	Clean with bleach	Weekly or more frequently
	Rinse glassware	Weekly
	Grease seals	Monthly
	Check calibration	Daily or when control is unsatisfactory
Centrifuge	Clean and disinfect	Weekly or more frequently
	Check speed	6-monthly
	Check times and locks	6-monthly
	Full maintenance	6-monthly
Temperature-controlled (water-baths, incubators, centrifuges, refrigerators)	Record upper and lower temperature extremes	Daily
Microscope	Full maintenance	6-monthly
Safety cabinet	Air flow	Weekly
	Full maintenance	6-monthly
pH meter	Two-point calibration	Daily
	Full maintenance	6-monthly
Pipettes	Calibrate	When first used
	Check tip	Each time used
Autodiluters/pipettes	Check calibration	Monthly
Photometers and spectrophotometers	Check calibration	Daily
	Prepare calibration graph	6-monthly
	Stability	*Ad-hoc*
	Full maintenance	6-monthly
Coagulometers	Check calibration	Daily
	Stability	*Ad-hoc*
	Full maintenance	6-monthly

The laboratory staff must ensure that equipment has been decontaminated in accordance with HN(87)22 when service or repair is required.

* Monitoring requirements vary among counters which have differing operating principles and degrees of automation.

identifying depletions and a means for triggering timely replacement. It must be closely monitored, regularly updated and kept sufficiently flexible to permit change. Allied to this is the provision of an appropriate storage environment (space, temperature, humidity, etc.) and a scheme to ensure that reagents are used in chronological order of reception within their specified shelf-lives. Contingency arrangements must be made for the purchase of small amounts of reagent in the event of failure of supply from the regular sources or to meet unexpected demand. Individual responsibility for these functions must be clearly identified. As a general principle the measures taken should ensure that a minimum of capital is invested in inventory and that wastage through out-dating is as low as possible.

Laboratory safety

For reasons of patient and staff safety the premises, where appropriate, should be divided into four procedural zones for patient reception, venesection, testing and administration. The following aspects of safety require specific consideration.

Microbial safety

General safety procedures must include sample manipulation, centrifugation, waste disposal, protective clothing and hygiene precautions (*Safe Working and the Prevention of Infection in Clinical Laboratories*, DHSS, 1990). Special consideration should be given to infectious specimens (ACDP, 1984) and those from patients in high risk groups—hepatitis B (Health Services Advisory Committee, 1985), HIV infection (ACDP, 1986) and viral haemorrhagic fevers (DHSS, 1986; ACDP, 1988). The policy for bacteriological assays should be clearly stated. General standards of hygiene must be enforced including prohibition of mouth pipetting, eating, smoking and the application of cosmetics in working areas. The importance of regular washing of hands must be stressed.

Various categories of clinical waste exist. Written procedures must describe disposal of each and staff must be trained in these methods (NCCLS, 1985). The laboratory is responsible for the supervision of disposal of various materials—(i) sharps, (ii) other disposables, (iii) non-disposables, including laundry, recycling of equipment and instruments.

If the laboratory is responsible for provision of a phlebotomy service, safety precautions must be defined for phlebotomists and included as part of their training.

Electrical safety

This includes both manufacturers' certification and procedures for installation and maintenance (DHSS, 1987, ESCHLE II).

Chemical hazards

(Health and Safety Commission, 1988).

Radiation hazards

(Health and Safety Commission, 1985).

Mechanical and other hazards

National guidelines for the handling of radioactive substances and the handling of samples from patients suspected of having hepatitis or HIV infections must be studied in detail and appropriate written individual laboratory codes of practice prepared.

All staff should be aware of safety precautions. All specimens should be treated as potentially infectious and should be handled in accordance with general rules of safety and the Code of Practice for prevention of infection in clinical laboratories and postmortem rooms (DHSS, 1978). Specimens from subjects who are known to be HIV antibody or HBsAg positive or who on clinical grounds are regarded as 'high risk' must be handled only by Senior MLSOs, approved scientific staff or medical staff in accordance with the relevant safety regulations.

Purchasing policy and maintenance contracts

All laboratory activities incur expense; however, in every case such expenditure may be controlled to some extent. Continuous cost control must be exercised to attain the effective balance between quality and cost of services. Quality at any price is unrealistic and must be substituted by the practice of cost effectiveness. As a primary event reliable procedural planning requiring detailed knowledge of certain key factors will permit rational assessment of 'best buy'. These factors include:

1 clinical need for a particular test and time demands
2 available personnel and premises
3 official product evaluation (both for instruments and kits)
4 availability of supplies
5 cost of supplies and equipment
6 details and conditions of warranty
7 'after sales' service including maintenance contracts.

The importance of maintenance contracts cannot be overestimated for the following reasons. First they contribute to cost savings by prolonging the life of instruments and additionally they result in the diminution of 'down-time'. Secondly, such maintenance of instruments contributes to overall quality assurance. Finally, any practice which reduces equipment malfunction with attendant hazard contributes to the safety and well-being of laboratory workers. Any contract should, in addition to cost and response time, specify what is included in and excluded from the service as well as identify the contact person.

Appendix: ICSH Definitions (ICSH Handbook 1986)

Standards

REFERENCE STANDARD

A substance or device, one or more properties of which are sufficiently well established to be used for the calibration of an apparatus, the assessment of a measurement method, or for assigning values to a material. Where possible it must be based on or traceable to exactly defined physical or chemical measurement.

INTERNATIONAL BIOLOGICAL STANDARDS

These are reference standards which cannot be determined by exactly defined physical or chemical measurement methods, but to which have been assigned international units of activity as defined by the World Health Organization. These materials are not intended to be used in the laboratory working procedures but serve as the means by which national and commercial reference materials and calibrators can be controlled.

Materials

REFERENCE METHOD

A clearly and exactly described technique for a particular determination which, in the opinion of a defined authority, provides sufficiently accurate and precise laboratory data for it to be used to assess the validity of other laboratory methods for this determination. The accuracy of the reference method must be established by comparison with a definitive method where one exists, and the degree of inaccuracy must be stated. The degree of imprecision must also be stated.

CALIBRATOR

A substance or device used to calibrate, graduate or adjust a measurement. It must be traceable to a reference standard (see 'Reference Standard' above).

CALIBRATION

The determination of a bias conversion factor of an analytical process under specified conditions, in order to obtain accurate measurement results. The accuracy over the operating range must be established by appropriate use of reference methods, reference materials and/or calibrators.

ACCURACY

A measure of agreement between the estimate of a value and the true value. Accuracy has no numerical value; it is measured as the amount of (degree of) inaccuracy.

INACCURACY

Numerical difference between the mean of a set of replicate measurements and the true value. This difference (positive or negative) may be expressed in the units in which the quantity is measured, or as a percentage of the true value.

BIAS

Systematic factor resulting in inaccuracy.

PRECISION

Agreement between replicate measurements. It has no numerical value but it is recognized in terms of imprecision.

IMPRECISION

Standard deviation or coefficient of variation of the results in a set of replicate measurements.

QUALITY CONTROL MATERIAL

A substance used in routine practice for checking the concurrent performance of an analytical process (or instrument). It must be similar in properties to and be analysed along with patient specimens. It may or may not have a pre-assigned value.

Quality assurance

QUALITY ASSURANCE PROGRAMMES

All steps to be taken by the director of a laboratory to ensure reliability of laboratory results and to increase accuracy, reproducibility and between-laboratory comparability. This includes proficiency surveillance (see below), the constant use of internal quality control and participation in an external quality assessment scheme. It also includes participation in training courses, conferences, collaborative studies of instruments and laboratory methods and other co-operative activities intended for the improvement of laboratory performance. A quality assurance programme in haematology must also be concerned with clinical aspects of haematology.

INTERNAL QUALITY CONTROL

Internal quality control is the set of procedures undertaken in a laboratory for the continual assessment of work carried out within the laboratory and evaluation of the results of tests to decide whether the latter are reliable enough to be released to the requesting clinician. The procedures should include tests on control material and statistical analysis of patients' data. The main object is to ensure day-to-day consistency of measurement or observation, if possible in agreement with an agreed indicator of truth such as control material with assigned values.

EXTERNAL QUALITY ASSESSMENT

External quality assessment refers to a system of retrospectively and objectively comparing results from different laboratories by means of surveys organized by an external agency. The main objective is to establish between-laboratory and between-instrument comparability, if possible in agreement with a reference standard where one exists. External quality assessment schemes may be regional, national or international. They may also be limited to the users of a particular instrument.

PROFICIENCY SURVEILLANCE

Supervision and action to ensure good laboratory practice. An important aspect is internal quality control and participation in an external quality assessment scheme, but it also includes attention to proficiency in specimen collection and labelling, delivery of specimens to the laboratory, record-keeping and reporting, environmental and storage effects on specimens, interpretation of test results and relevance of various tests for the clinical information required. It also includes maintenance and control of equipment and apparatus, staff training and protection of staff health and safety.

References

AABB (1981) *Standards for blood banks and transfusion services.* American Association of Blood Banks, Washington D.C., USA.

ACDP (Advisory Committee on Dangerous Pathogens), (1984) *Categorisation of pathogens according to hazard and categories of containment.* HMSO.

ACDP (Advisory Committee on Dangerous Pathogens), (1990) Second Revision of Guidelines—*The Causative Agent of AIDS and related Conditions*—HMSO.

ACDP (Advisory Committee on Dangerous Pathogens), (1988) *Inactivation of viral haemorrhagic fever specimens with β-propriololactins.* HMSO.

Department of Trade and Industry, (1987) *Guide to the Consumer Protection Act 1987, Product Liability and Safety Provisions.* HMSO.

DHSS (1978) *Code of Practice for the Prevention of Infection in Clinical Laboratories and Post-Mortem Rooms (The 'Howie Code of Practice').* HMSO.

DHSS (1986) *Memorandum on the Control of Viral Haemorrhagic Fevers.* HMSO.

DHSS (1987) *Electrical Safety Code for Hospital Laboratory Equipment (ESCHLE)* 2nd edn. Health Equipment Information No. 158.

DHSS (1987) HN(87)22, *Decontamination of Health Care Equipment Prior to Inspection, Service or Repair.*

DHSS (1988) HN(88)3, HN(FP)[88]5, *Procurement Product Liability.*

Health and Safety Commission (1975) *Health and Safety at Work Act 1974, Advice to Employers (HSC 3).* HMSO.

Health and Safety Commission (1985) *The Protection of Persons Against Ionising Radiation Arising from any Work Practice.* Approved Code of Practice, HMSO.

Health and Safety Commission (1988) *Control of Substances Hazardous to Health.* COSHH Regulations, Approved Codes of Practice, HMSO.

Health Services Advisory Committee (1985) *Safety in Health Service Laboratories: Hepatitis B.* HMSO.

Holburn, A.M. (1982) Quality Assurance and Standardization in blood group serology. In Cavill I. (ed.) *Methods in Haematology Quality Control*, pp. 34–50. Churchill Livingstone, Edinburgh.

Hoppe, A.H. (1979) *Considerations in the selection of reagents.* Appendix 1:15. American Association of Blood Banks, Washington.

ICSH (International Committee for Standardisation in Haematology) (1981) The Theory of Reference Values. *Clinical and Laboratory Haematology*, **3**, 369–373.

ICSH (International Committee for Standardisation in Haematology) (1984) Protocol for Evaluation of Automated Blood Cell Counters. *Clinical and Laboratory Haematology* **6**, 69–84.

ICSH (International Committee for Standardisation in Haematology) (1986) *Rules and Operating Procedures Handbook.*

NCCLS (National Committee for Clinical Laboratory Standards) (1985) *Clinical Laboratory Hazardous Waste.* Proposed Guideline Document GP5-P. Vol. 6, NCCLS, Villanova, PA, USA.

Voak, D. & Napier J.A.F. (1990) Quality Assurance in the Hospital Transfusion Laboratory: Quality Control in Blood Group Serology. In Cavill I. (ed.) *Methods in Haematology Quality Control* 2nd edn, pp. 129–153. Churchill Livingstone, Edinburgh.

2 Role of the Blood Film with Automated Blood Counting Systems

Prepared by the
General Haematology Task Force

When the haemoglobin concentration and packed cell volume are known, a reliable diagnosis of most blood disorders can be made by examining a blood film microscopically. In recent years the introduction of automated blood cell counters has resulted in the inclusion of a number of other parameters in the blood count. These are measured with remarkable precision and speed, thus allowing a significant increase in the number of blood examinations that can be carried out and at relatively low cost for what had previously been a labour-intensive series of tests. Automated instruments for blood counting range from fairly simple instruments which count red cells or leucocytes in a sample of blood which has been prediluted manually, to systems which perform the blood count, including a full differential count, as well as red cell and platelet size distribution analyses in less than 1 minute from an automatically aspirated sample of whole blood.

In most haematology laboratories the workload continues to increase year by year, especially for 'routine' blood counts, and only by means of these automated systems can the laboratories meet the demand. It is a haematological tradition that microscopic examination of the stained peripheral blood smear is an important adjunct to the blood count. This ideal is no longer practical and, clearly, film scrutiny is not necessary in all instances. Laboratories adopt different strategies in deciding which films to examine and on which of these to perform a full differential leucocyte count (DLC). This decision is generally based on the clinical history, the immediate blood count results, and the previous results. There is, however, little published information on practice. In a survey, (Lewis, unpublished observations), conducted in 1988 in the UK by the National External Quality Assessment Scheme (NEQAS), data from 422 UK laboratories revealed that 23×10^6 blood count requests were made annually. Of the laboratories analysed, 53% (222) were using automated counters: 215 were flow cytometers (134 performing three-part DLC and 81 a five-part) and seven image analysis instruments. Blood films were examined in every case in 18 laboratories

Working Party: A.J. Birch, M. Brozović, S.M. Lewis, R.M. Rowan, N.K. Shinton.

but in the rest only when indicated by clinical or instrument flag. Overall, in some 25% of the tests was blood film examination performed. However, this is a rapidly changing situation as an increasing number of laboratories are using counters of various levels of automation, including the fully automated blood cell analysers. This, together with reduction in the numbers of medical and technical staff available to undertake blood film examination, makes it timely to assess the need for blood film examination in the routine haematology service.

The essential question to be considered is the reliability of the counters to identify abnormalities which would have been detected on the blood film and conversely the reliability of the blood film and the comparability between instrument-derived quantitative measurements and subjective impressions, by an observer, of macrocytosis, hypochromasia, etc.

The precision and low CV of total erythrocytes, leucocytes and platelet counts has been well demonstrated with most of the instruments on the market today including the simpler, less costly machines. The accuracy of these counters is less easily assessed as there are few standards available and comparison is generally made with selected routine methods. Differences between instruments are found when comparing cell volumes, especially the mean erythrocyte volume (MCV) and the mean platelet volume (MPV). The ability of instrument microprocessors to analyse cell size distribution has led to the introduction of new measurements of dispersion—red cell distribution width (RDW) and platelet distribution width (PDW). Unfortunately, different machines use different methods of calculation for the RDW, thus causing confusion. Bessman *et al.* (1983) proposed a comprehensive classification of anaemias based on RDW–MCV results but a review by Simel (1987) concluded that this classification was of value in primary care only as an aid to differentiation of iron deficiency from thalassaemia.

RDW and PDW are quantitative expressions of anisocytosis of red cells and platelets respectively; MCV and MCHC express red cell size and haemoglobin concentrations. Undoubtedly, instruments are reliable, more so than the human eye, in measuring degrees of hypochromasia and in distinguishing borderline macrocytosis or microcytosis. On the other hand machines are unlikely to detect schistocytes, basophilic stippling, Howell–Jolly bodies, Heinz bodies, nucleated red cells or malarial parasites. Rouleaux of erythrocytes cannot be detected by machine. With some instruments certain abnormal red cells may react atypically with the diluent reagents, leading to false measurements. This occurs especially with haemoglobinopathies which are resistant to sphering, whilst malarial parasites may confuse the instrument into giving false values for lymphocytes.

Continuous flow cytochemistry using Hemalog D (Technicon) was claimed to be of value in recognizing acute leukaemia, in distinguishing acute lymphoblastic (ALL) and acute myeloblastic (AML) leukaemias, and in differentiating subgroups of AML (Patterson *et al.*, 1980; Hinchcliffe *et al.*, 1981; d'Onofrio &

Mango, 1984). This instrument was replaced by the H-6000 and Lai *et al.* (1986) compared the two instruments with S-Plus IV (Coulter) for the diagnosis of ALL and AML. They found that all three machines were highly effective in recognizing the presence of an abnormality and all were of value in distinguishing AML from ALL. However, the presence in some cases of AML of large numbers of micromyeloblasts recognized as 'lymphocytes' limited the discriminating power of all three machines. Definition of sub-types of AML was not possible. In a further study of chronic lymphocytic leukaemia (CLL) and hairy cell leukaemia (HCL) (Lai *et al.*, 1987) the three machines detected 'lymphocytosis', Hemalog D and H-6000 also detecting monocytopenia in HCL and raised numbers of large unstained cells (LUC) in CLL.

Reports on other machines have been less satisfactory. Cross and Strange (1987) reported erroneous results in CLL when using ELT 800/WS. Allen (1988) found that the Coulter S Plus IV leucocyte volume analysis has acceptable limits of operation for detection of blasts while not being specific.

Blood film screening does not necessarily include a differential leucocyte count, but this must be considered in the context of the 'blood count'. In general, automated instruments have been shown to be reliable in a two-part differential count, for distinguishing neutrophils and lymphocytes, but less reliable in classifying monocytes, eosinophils and basophils, as required for the traditional five-part differential count. Also, as described above, whilst some instruments can flag blasts and other abnormal cells in the blood, this is not consistent and they are unlikely to give the overall diagnostic information that can be obtained from a blood film. The question therefore arises as to when a blood film should be examined as a supplement to the automated count and DLC. Can a normal automated count be used as a means of exclusion, and what flags should be used for inclusion? A flagging system has been devised by Koepke *et al.* (1985) and algorithms have been proposed by Dutcher (1985).

Claims have been made for equivalent sensitivity of machine with microscopic differential counting (Richardson-Jones *et al.*, 1985). Comparison of 3,500 specimens using the Coulter S Plus IV machine with microscopy showed a false negative rate of $< 4\%$, these being due to eosinophilia, increased 'band' forms and a few atypical lymphocytes, and a false positive rate of 30% (Rappaport *et al.*, 1988). A microcomputer programme developed by McClure *et al.* (1988) analysed the numeric data from a machine with 156 predominantly abnormal subjects, 200 predominantly normal subjects and 200 normal subjects and compared the outcome with a set of criteria for morphological examination developed by Payne and Pierre (1986). The computer programme was more sensitive for bands, immature granulocytes, monocytes, nucleated erythrocytes, reticulocytosis, poikilocytosis, schistocytosis, and hypersegmented neutrophils whereas the numerical data was more sensitive for eosinophilia.

The reports which follow are based on current UK practice in which the blood film has had an important role in diagnostic haematology. Algorithms are proposed to allow the continuation of this practice despite large workloads in the diagnostic service, by means of selective use of the blood film integrated with measurements by Coulter S Plus IV, Sysmex E5000 and Technicon H*1 or H-6000, respectively. The utility of the algorithms and their validity when linked to the particular counters may not necessarily apply to other counters or to other working practices. The procedures used to validate the algorithms should however serve as a model to construct an algorithm for a particular situation.

References

Allen B.C. (1988) Coulter Plus IV leucocyte volume analysis instrument: sensitivity of blast identification in peripheral blood. *Journal of Clinical Pathology* **41**, 1136–1137.

Bessman, J.D., Gilmer P.R. & Gardner F.H. (1983) Improved classification of anaemia by MCV and RDW. *American Journal of Clinical Pathology* **80**, 322–326.

Cross J. & Strange C.A. (1987) Erroneous Ortho ELT 800/WS WBC in chronic lymphatic leukaemia. *Clinical and Laboratory Haematology* **9**, 371–376.

d'Onofrio G. & Mango, G. (1984) Automated cytochemistry in acute leukaemia. *Acta Haematologica* **72**, 221–230.

Dutcher T.F. (1985) Automated differentials: a strategy *Blood Cells* **11**, 49–59.

Hinchcliffe R.F., Lilleyman J.S., Burrows N.F. & Swan H.T. (1981) Use of the Hemalog D automated leucocyte differential counter in the diagnosis and therapy of leukaemia. *Acta Haematologica* **65**, 79–84.

Koepke J., Dotson M.A., Shifman M.W. & Boyarski M.W. (1985) A flagging system for multichannel haematology analysers. *Blood Cells* **11**, 113–126.

Lai A.P., Martin P.J., Richards J.D.M., Goldstone A.M. & Cawley J.C. (1986) Automated leucocyte differential counts in acute leukaemia: a comparison of the Hemalog D, H6000 and Coulter S Plus IV. *Clinical and Laboratory Haematology* **8**, 33–42.

Lai A.P., Martin P.J., Cawley J.D., Richards J.D.M. & Goldstone A.M. (1987) Automated leucocyte differential counts in chronic lymphatic and hairy cell leukaemias: a comparison of Hemalog D, H6000 and Coulter S Plus IV. *Clinical and Laboratory Haematology* **9**, 169–174.

McClure S., Bates J.E., Harrison R., Gilmer P.R. & Bessman J.D. (1988) The 'Diff-If'. *American Journal of Clinical Pathology* **90**, 163–168.

Martin P.J., Anderson C.C., Jones H.M., Lai A.P., Linch D.C. & Goldstone A.H. (1986) A rise in the percentage of large unstained cells in the peripheral blood determined by the Hemalog D90 automated differential counter is a feature of impending myeloid engraftment following bone marrow transplantation. *Clinical and Laboratory Haematology* **8**, 1–8.

Patterson K.G., Cawley J.C., Goldstone A.H., Richards J.D.M. & Janossy G. (1980) A comparison of automated cytochemical analysis and conventional methods in the classification of acute leukaemia. *Clinical and Laboratory Haematology* **2**, 281–291.

Payne B.A. & Pierre R.V. (1986) Using the three part differential. *Laboratory Medicine* **17**, 459–462 and 517–522.

Rappaport E.S., Helbert B., Beissner R.S. & Trowbridge A. (1988) Automated hematology: where we stand. *Southern Medical Journal* **81**, 365–370.

Richardson-Jones A., Hellman R. & Twedt (1985) The Coulter counter leucocyte differential. *Blood Cells* **11**, 203–240.

Simel D.L. (1987) Review: is the RDW-MCV classification of anaemia useful? *Clinical and Laboratory Haematology* **9**, 349–360.

3 Assessment of the Need for Blood Film Examination with Blood Counts by Second Generation Light Scatter Counters

Prepared by the General Haematology Task Force

The study describes the efficacy of using a selection procedure combined with second generation light scatter counters in reducing the proportion of films examined microscopically. Four laboratories participated, three with H-6000 and one with H-1 Technicon cell counters. Each laboratory used its own procedure to select films for microscopy. The number of films examined was reduced by 40–80% depending on the local procedure. The automated count and differential were considered to be inadequate in only 1.6% of specimens where the films were predicted to be normal and not examined by the routine screener. In contrast, between 9 and 32% of specimens categorized as 'in need of microscopic examination', were in fact normal. The sensitivity of the selection procedure with the H-6000 counters was 68%, and with the H-1 counter was 83%. Their specificities were 76% and 55% respectively, with a positive predictive value of 66% and 42.0%, and a negative predictive value of 79% and 89% for the H-6000 and the H-1 counters. All four laboratories were reliable in predicting normality, but less successful in predicting abnormality. Certain morphological abnormalities can only be detected visually.

Introduction

The introduction of automated blood cell differential counting has reduced the necessity for microscopic blood film examination. Claims have been made for the effectiveness of continuous flow cytometry in the detection of acute leukaemia (Patterson *et al.*, 1980; Hinchcliffe *et al.*, 1981; d'Onofrio & Mango, 1984; Lai *et al.*, 1986), hairy cell leukaemia (Lai *et al.*, 1987) and detection of myeloid engraftment following bone marrow transplantation (Martin *et al.*, 1986). An atlas comparing automated flow cytometry histograms with blood films (Simson *et al.*, 1988) suggests that the microscopic examination has been superseded by the automated machine. Furthermore, automated machines increase throughput and reduce the cost per test. The need for microscopic blood film examination

Working Party: A.J. Birch, M. Brozović, S.M. Lewis, R.M. Rowan, N.K. Shinton.

must therefore be considered, and any method of selection for microscopic scrutiny assessed. Can a normal automated count and differential be used as a means of exclusion, and what indicators or flags should be used for inclusion?

The present study was devised to establish the efficacy of the selection procedure used with the second generation light scatter differential counters in four laboratories in selecting blood films for examination. We attempted to establish whether it was practical and safe to examine visually blood films from a proportion of specimens only.

Design of the study

Four laboratories participated; three are in large district general hospitals, and the fourth is in a teaching hospital with many specialized units. The teaching hospital laboratory used H-1; the other three used H-6000 counters. The study was initiated in 1986 and completed in 1987.

A total of 4007 specimens was examined. Each laboratory included the specimens from at least one haematology outpatient clinic. The percentage of 'haematology' samples varied between 12.0 and 33.3.

The design is shown in Figure 3.1. Each laboratory followed its own procedure for selecting specimens for microscopic examination by the routine screener. During the study period (7 to 14 days), a proforma was completed for each specimen received by the laboratory. Films were made on all specimens, but only films on specimens which fulfilled the criteria for microscopic examination by the routine screener were looked at. The comments were entered on the proforma. At a later date, a local referee examined all the blood films from the study period regardless of whether or not they had already been looked at

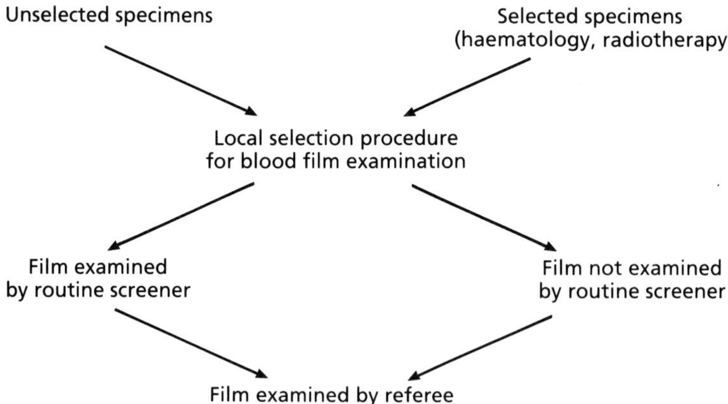

Fig. 3.1 Design of the study.

'routinely'. The referee's comments were also entered on the proforma. The proformata were analysed as described in the Results section.

Three categories or flags were used to decide whether or not to examine a film:

1 Clinical flag: patient category, age, diagnosis, type of treatment, etc. Clinical flags differed between the laboratories as shown in Table 3.1.

2 Instrumental flag: numerical result outside the laboratory reference range, abnormal red cell or platelet indices, wider than normal (for the laboratory) red cell histogram, abnormal shape or position of the leukocyte cloud, abnormal machine differential, HPX, presence of platelet clumps or suspected nucleated red cells, etc.

3 Delta check flag: two laboratories with cumulative reporting flagged any result which showed a significant (as defined locally) difference from the previous one. This included changes in blood count, indices and differential.

The distribution of specimens according to these criteria at the different laboratories are shown in Figures 3.2, 3.3 and 3.4.

Results

The failure or success of the selection procedure was assessed by the number of 'abnormal' and 'normal' films in each of the four categories shown in Table 3.2. A normal film was defined as the film on which the referee made either no comment, or commented 'normal film' or 'no abnormality detected'. An abnormal film was defined as any film where the referee made any comment other

Table 3.1 Clinical selection or 'clinical flag' criteria for the four laboratories

Laboratory 1	Specific 'haematology' requests Clinical diagnosis of glandular fever or PUO Recent visit to Africa or Asia
Laboratory 2	Haematological malignancies Patients with enlarged lymph nodes, liver or spleen Clinical diagnosis of glandular fever or PUO Patients with bleeding diathesis Patients with sickle cell disease in crisis Requests for parasites
Laboratory 3	Haematology clinic patients Requests for film, reticulocytes, platelets or parasites 'Listed' diagnoses
Laboratory 4	Diagnosed blood disease patients Neonates Patients receiving radiotherapy or chemotherapy Other patients, when indicated by clinical information (chronic renal failure, infectious mononucleosis etc.)

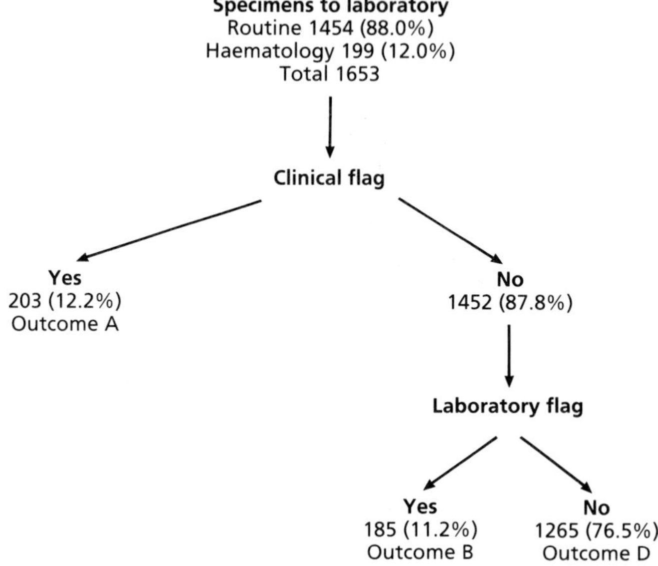

Fig. 3.2 Decision chart for laboratories 1 and 2.

Table 3.2 Concordance between prediction and microscopic scrutiny

			% total		
Set	Prediction	Referee	1 + 2	3	4
True positives	Abnormal	Abnormal	14.1	41.3	23.1
True negatives	Normal	Normal	67.8	28.8	40.3
False positives	Abnormal	Normal	9.1	16.6	31.8
False negatives	Normal	Abnormal	8.8	13.3	4.8

Laboratories 1, 2 and 3 are in district general hospitals, laboratory 4 is in a teaching hospital. The results from laboratories 1 and 2 are combined because their selection procedures were almost identical.

than ‘normal film’ or ‘no abnormality detected’. The four categories were defined according to Galen and Gambino (1975).

1 True positives or true abnormals, where both the prediction and the microscopic examination by the referee showed an abnormality.

2 True negatives or true normals, where the prediction and the microscopic examination by the referee agreed on normality.

3 False positives or false abnormals, where the film was predicted to be abnormal, but found to be normal by the referee.

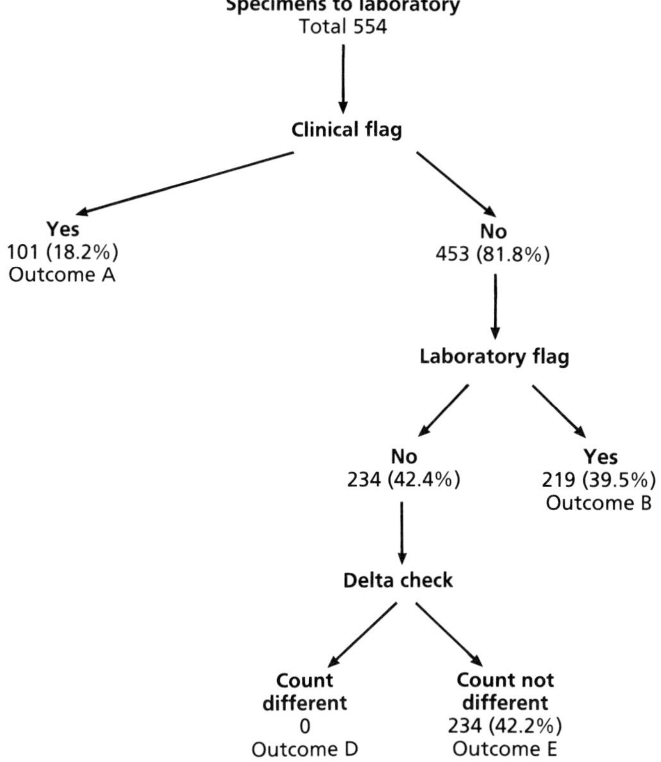

Fig. 3.3 Decision chart for laboratory 3.

4 False negatives or false normals, where the film was predicted to be normal but found to be abnormal by the referee.

If the selection procedure were ideal all specimens would fall into the category of either true positives or true negatives. As can be seen from Table 3.2, the percentage of false negatives varied between 4.8 and 13.3. The percentage of false positives ranged between 9.1 and 31.8.

The sensitivity (percentage of films found to be abnormal by the local referee, amongst those predicted to be abnormal and routinely examined), specificity (percentage of films found to be normal by the referee, amongst those predicted to be normal and not examined by the routine screener), the predictive value of abnormality and of normality are shown in Table 3.3. It must be emphasized that the sensitivity and specificity reflect not only the instrument performance but also the characteristics of each laboratory's selection procedure and the idiosyncrasies of the local referee. Furthermore, predictive values reflect the proportion of abnormal specimens in each hospital.

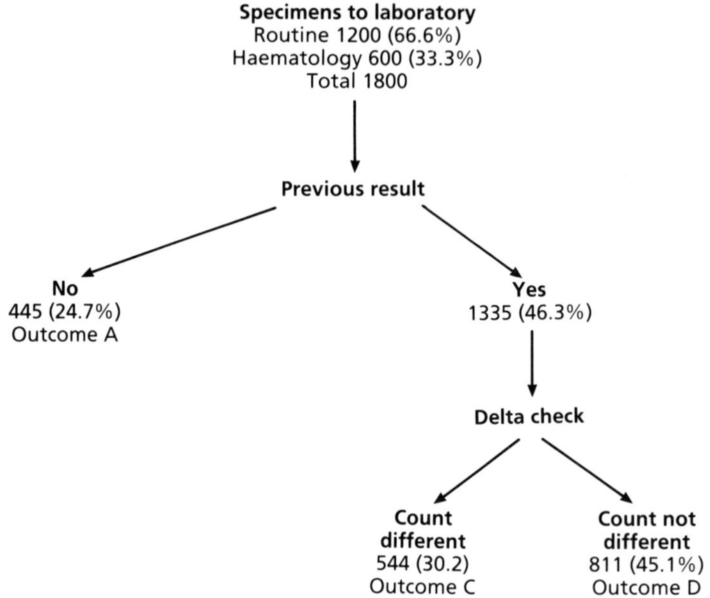

Outcomes A and C, films examined = 989 (54.9%). Out of 445 specimens in outcome A 243 (13.5%) showed an instrumental flag, whereas 202 (11.2%) were 'normal'.
Outcome D, films were not examined = 811 (45.1%).

Fig. 3.4 Decision chart for laboratory 4.

Table 3.3 Predictive values for the four laboratories

			Predictive value (%) of:	
Laboratory	Sensitivity %	Specificity %	Films routinely examined for abnormality	Films not examined routinely for normality
1 + 2	61.8	88.7	60.8	88.7
3	75.4	63.4	71.2	68.3
4	82.9	55.4	42.0	89.2
Overall	73.3	65.5	58.0	82.0

The concordance between the instrument and the manual differential (Table 3.4) was assessed on the basis of the number of inadequate differentials: an inadequate differential was defined by each referee as the differential where the disagreement between the instrumental and the visual differential was of sufficient magnitude to warrant discarding the instrumental one. Of the films predicted to be normal (total of 2310) 37 or 1.6% were considered to be inadequate, whereas amongst those predicted to be abnormal (total of 1697), 160 or 9.4% were considered to be inadequate by the referee (Table 3.5). The reasons

Table 3.4 Concordance between the referee and the instrumental differential

Laboratory	Concordance %
1 + 2	98.5
3	93.7
4	92.2
Overall % of instrumental differentials considered concordant by the referee	94.8

Table 3.5 Inadequate differentials by prediction category according to referees

	Inadequate instrument differentials amongst:			
	Predicted normal films		Predicted abnormal films	
Laboratory	No.	%	No.	%
1 + 2	1	0.07	23	5.9
3	6	2.5	31	9.9
4	30	3.7	105	10.6
Overall	37	1.6	159	9.3

for inadequate differentials varied and are shown in Table 3.6: blasts were missed in 16 specimens, but all were in known leukaemics whose films had been predicted to be abnormal. The single largest category of inadequate differentials was caused by the failure of the H-6000 to detect left shift and the spurious left shift flagged by the H-1. All machine differentials in chronic phase CGL, myelofibrosis and leukoerythroblastic anaemias were considered inadequate. Spurious eosinophilia and basophilia were found in 23 specimens. Five abnormal

Table 3.6 Reasons for inadequate differentials according to referees

Reasons	H-6000	H-1
Failure to detect blasts	8	8
Failure to detect left shift	26	0
Spurious left shift	0	83
Spurious basophilia	4	6
Spurious eosinophilia	0	11
Failure to detect other white cell abnormalities*	7	21
Spurious white cell abnormalities†	5	7
Other‡	8	0
Total	60	136

* Monocytosis, atypical mononuclears, hairy cells, eosinophilia, lymphocytosis.

† Myeloperoxidase deficiency, monocytosis, neutropenia, abnormal shape of the leukocyte cloud, etc.

‡ Nucleated red cells, EDTA changes, platelet clumps.

differentials were due to myeloperoxidase deficiency: they were normal on microscopy of Giemsa stained films.

The combined value of all inadequate differentials gives a measure of the overall concordance between the microscopic and instrumental differential as shown in Table 3.4. The very high concordance in laboratories 1 and 2 is also a reflection of their workload which contained many normal specimens sent from the community.

An attempt to assess the usefulness of the selection procedure and the counter in providing the information on the morphological appearances of the blood film was made through the analysis of the comments made by the referees (Table 3.7). The number of films commented upon was higher (as expected) in the category predicted to be abnormal than in the predicted normals.

The analysis of red cell and white cell comments (Tables 3.8 and 3.9) confirms the inability of machines to flag certain abnormalities, such as rouleaux, polychromasia, target cells, red cell fragments, hypersegmented polymorphs, hypograndular neutrophils, atypical mononuclears and many others. The referees were not asked to comment on the clinical significance of these machine 'misses' and it is therefore impossible to assess how much clinically relevant information may have been lost in the films not examined microscopically. Some comments, such as poikilocytosis, target cells and right shift were more common in laboratories 1 and 2, than in laboratory 3. This may reflect a true difference (a large ethnic population with many heterozygotes for haemoglobin abnormalities) or the local referee's idiosyncrasies. The majority of referee comments appeared with similar frequencies in different specimen categories (routinely visually examined or not) and in different laboratories.

Discussion

The study confirms that, with a judicious use of a selection procedure, it is possible to reduce the number of films examined visually with minimal risk of missing serious pathology. Such a selection procedure must be devised with the

Table 3.7 Analysis of comments (other than 'normal film') made by referees

	Films predicted abnormal commented		Films predicted normal commented		Total commented	
Laboratory	No.	%	No.	%	No.	%
1 + 2	236	60.8	146	11.5	382	24.4
3	228	71.2	74	31.6	308	55.5
4	416	42.1	87	10.7	503	27.9
Total	880	51.8	307	13.2	1193	29.7

Table 3.8 Analysis of red cell comments made by the referees

	Laboratory			
	1 + 2		3	
	Not examined routinely	Examined routinely	Not examined routinely	Examined routinely
Total no. of films	1265	386	234	320
No. of films commented upon by the referee	146	236	74	228
Comments				
Polychromasia	32 (21.9)*	53 (22.4)	5 (6.7)	31 (13.5)
Dimorphic	38 (26.0)	32 (21.9)	6 (8.1)	35 (15.3)
Poikilocytosis	102 (71.0)	70 (47.9)	6 (8.1)	44 (19.2)
Elliptocytosis	3 (2.0)	2 (0.8)	1 (1.3)	2 (0.7)
Pencil forms	14 (9.5)	11 (4.6)	0	14 (6.1)
Target cells	22 (15.1)	50 (21.1)	1 (1.3)	19 (8.3)
Echinocytes	30 (20.8)	16 (6.7)	2 (2.7)	3 (1.3)
Acanthocytes	2 (1.3)	0	4 (5.4)	4 (1.7)
Burr cells	9 (6.1)	6 (2.5)	2 (2.7)	18 (7.9)
Fragments	26 (10.9)	19 (8.0)	0	0
Sickle cells	0	16 (6.7)	0	0
Stomatocytes	0	0	9 (12.1)	0
Ovalocytes	0	4 (1.6)	5 (6.7)	13 (5.7)
Spherocytes	0	1 (0.4)	0	1 (1.3)
Rouleaux	74 (50.6)	32 (13.5)	24 (32.4)	83 (36.4)
Agglutination	1 (0.6)	4 (1.6)	1 (1.3)	0
Howell–Jolly bodies	0	9 (3.8)	0	7 (3.0)
Punctate basophilia	0	0	0	0
Parasites	0	0	0	0

* Figures in parentheses express results as a percentage.

specific problems of the individual laboratory in mind; the type and the size of the workload, as well as the cost per test and staffing considerations. District general hospitals will probably be able to reduce the number of films examined to 20–30%. This is unlikely to be the case in the teaching hospitals or hospitals with renal, radiotherapy and other specialized units.

It must, however, be accepted that machines cannot flag certain morphological abnormalities, such as rouleaux, poikilocytosis, red cell fragments, parasites, or finer changes in white cells. Neither can they distinguish reliably between different immature white cells. Nevertheless, the concordance between the instrumental differential and the visual one is excellent and was over 92% in all four laboratories.

The sensitivity of 73.3% is lower than the 83.8% reported by Kline *et al.* in 1989 as shown by the number of missing 'blasts' in 16 of the 4007 samples examined. The specificity of only 65.5% is also less than their finding of 78.9%

Table 3.9 Analysis of white cell comments made by the referees

	Laboratory			
	1 + 2		3	
	Not examined routinely	Examined routinely	Not examined routinely	Examined routinely
Total no. of films	1265	386	234	320
No. of films commented upon by the referee	146	236	74	228
Right shift	22 (15.0)*	35 (14.8)	1 (1.1)	11 (4.8)
Left shift	12 (8.2)	23 (14.8)	7 (9.4)	29 (12.7)
Pelger abnormality	0	1 (0.4)	0	0
Vacuolation	5 (3.4)	3 (1.2)	1 (1.3)	1 (0.3)
Toxic granulation	46 (31.5)	26 (11.0)	9 (12.7)	34 (14.9)
Dohle bodies	1 (0.6)	2 (0.8)	0	1 (0.3)
Hypogranularity	7 (4.7)	3 (1.2)	0	2 (0.7)
Hairy cells	0	1 (0.4)	0	1 (0.3)
Smear cells	0	2 (0.8)	1 (1.3)	11 (14.8)
Atypical mononuclears	2 (1.3)	7 (2.9)	1 (1.3)	0
Reactive lymphocytes	6 (4.1)	32 (13.5)	11 (14.8)	11 (14.8)
Cleft nuclei	0	6 (2.5)	0	0
Plasma cells	0	2 (0.8)	0	0
Auer rods	0	2 (0.8)	0	0

* Figures in parentheses express results as a percentage.

but their report did not include non-leukaemic patients. Our results are also contrary to the findings of Lai *et al.* (1986) whose machines detected all 32 known cases of acute leukaemia. It follows that the reliability depends on the selection procedure set for the laboratory: the higher the percentage of the films examined the less likely it is to miss significant pathology. This is confirmed in our study: laboratory 4 had the highest sensitivity and the lowest number of false normals, but they also had the highest number of false abnormals!

No selection procedure is fool proof, but an intelligent balance between the minimum risk and the maximum laboratory efficiency should be sought. The implementation of such a selection policy will inevitably result in the loss of some morphological information which is only available through visual inspection. The importance of the 'lost' morphology must be judged for each laboratory individually and depends on the type of workload, staffing, and local expectations.

References

d'Onofrio G. & Mango G. (1984) Automated cytochemistry in acute leukaemia. *Acta Haematologica* **72**, 221–230.

Galen R.S. & Gambino S.R. (1975) *Beyond normality: The predictive value and efficiency of medical diagnosis*. John Wiley, New York.

Hinchcliffe R.M., Lilleyman J.S., Burrows N.F. & Swan H.T. (1981) Use of the Hemalog D automated leukocyte differential counter in the diagnosis and therapy of leukaemia. *Acta Haematologica* **65**, 79–84.

Kawarabayashi K., Tsidi I., Tatsumi N., Okunda K. (1987) Leukemic blasts detected by the H-1 blood counter. *American Journal of Clinical Pathology* **88**, 624–627.

Kline A., Bird A., Adams A., Wale C., Edwards F. & Pereira E. (1989) Identification of blast cells in the peripheral blood of patients with acute leukaemia using Technicon H-1, *Clinical and Laboratory Haematology* **11**, 111–116.

Lai A.P., Martin P.J., Richards J.D.M., Goldstone A.M. & Cawley J.C. (1986) Automated leukocyte differential counts in acute leukaemia: a comparison of Hemalog D, H-6000 and Coulter S-Plus IV. *Clinical and Laboratory Haematology* **8**, 33–42.

Lai A.P., Martin P.J., Cawley J.D., Richards J.D.M. & Goldstone A.H. (1987) Automated leukocyte differential counts in chronic lymphatic and hairy cell leukaemias: a comparison of Hemalog D, H-6000 and Coulter S-Plus IV. *Clinical and Laboratory Haematology* **9**, 169–174.

Martin P.J., Anderson C.C., Jones H.M., Lai A.P., Linch D.C. & Goldstone A.H. (1986) A rise in the percentage of large unstained cells in the peripheral blood determined by the Hemalog D90 automated differential counter is a feature of impending myeloid engraftment following bone marrow transplantation. *Clinical and Laboratory Haematology* **8**, 1–8.

Patterson K.G., Cawley J.C., Goldstone A.H., Richards J.D.M. & Janossy G. (1980) A comparison of automated cytochemical analysis and conventional methods in the classification of acute leukaemia. *Clinical and Laboratory Haematology* **2**, 281–291.

Rappaport E.S., Helbert B., Beissner R.S. & Trowbridge A. (1988) Automated haematology: where we stand. *Southern Medical Journal* **81**, 365–370.

Simson E., Ross D.W. & Kocher W.D. (1988) *Atlas of Automated Cytochemical Hematology*. Technicon Instruments Corporation, New York.

4 Assessment of the Need for Blood Film Examination with Blood Counts by Aperture–Impedance Systems

Prepared by the
General Haematology Task Force

To meet the needs of present-day practice critical selection of blood films for scrutiny is necessary as a back-up to automated blood counts. An algorithm has been proposed in which the categories of cases requiring blood films are defined. In order to assess the utility of the algorithm, a study has been carried out with two different instruments (Coulter S Plus IV and Sysmex [Toa] E5000) at two teaching hospitals with specialized haematology units. It was possible to reduce the number of films by 30–40% without serious effect on blood count reliability although a small number of abnormal features of possible clinical relevance might then be missed. The counters performed similarly with a sensitivity of 95%, a specificity of 81%, a positive predictive value of 74%, a negative predictive value of 96% and overall efficiency of 85%.

Introduction

The workload in most haematology laboratories continues to increase year by year, especially for 'routine' blood counts. It is a haematological tradition that microscopic examination of the stained peripheral blood smear is an important adjunct to measuring the various components of the blood count. This ideal is no longer practical and, clearly, blood film scrutiny is not necessary in all instances. Laboratories adopt different strategies in deciding which films to examine and on which of these to perform a full differential leucocyte count (DLC). This decision is generally based on the clinical history, the immediate blood count results, and the previous results. There is no doubt that computerized data storage greatly assists this procedure.

In a survey conducted in 1988 in the UK by the National External Quality Assessment Scheme (NEQAS), data from some 422 UK laboratories revealed that 23×10^6 FBC requests are made annually. Of the laboratories analysed, 53% (222) were using automated counters: 215 flow cytometers (134 performing a three-part DLC and 81 a five-part) and 7 image analysis instruments. Blood films

Working Party: S.M. Lewis, R.M. Rowan.

were examined in every case in 18 laboratories but only when indicated by clinical or instrument flag in the remainder. Overall, blood film examination was performed in some 25% of the tests. However, this is a rapidly changing situation as most laboratories are now using counters of various levels of automation, with an increasing number of fully automated blood cell analysers which include measurements of red cell and platelet size and size distribution coupled with varying components of the differential white cell count. Relative (and absolute) reduction in the numbers of medical and technical staff available to undertake microscopy makes it timely to assess the need for blood film examination in the routine haematology service.

There have been no detailed investigations on the utility of aperture–impedance instruments for distinguishing which specimens merit a blood film examination and which do not. The present study has attempted to answer this question in relation to the Coulter Counter Model S Plus IV (aperture–impedance with electronic editing) and the Toa (Sysmex) E5000 (aperture–impedance with sheathed flow).

Design of study

While the basic design is similar to that described in the preceding chapter (see Fig. 3.1) for routinely selecting specimens for microscopic examination, the main thrust of the present study is to evaluate the adequacy of the instruments to recognize abnormality rather than the efficacy and safety of the flow chart.

The study was undertaken in the diagnostic laboratories of two large teaching hospital haematology departments. A Coulter Counter Model S Plus IV was used in one (Hospital 1) and a Sysmex (Toa) E5000 in the other (Hospital 2).

The study was designed to assess how often the instruments' numerical results, graphical displays and/or flags could replace the need for microscopy; how often a false positive flag appeared and the impact this had on workload; and finally how often a false negative result emerged and the impact this had on patient management. The two hospitals are major centres with numerous special units; thus, the haematological practice and the need for blood film examination to satisfy diagnostic requirements might be expected to be similar, but to differ from the situation in a district general hospital. Flow charts for determining the need for blood film examination were designed for both laboratories. As these differed only in very minor detail a single algorithm was proposed which was considered to be suitable for use in either establishment (Fig. 4.1).

According to this, blood films would be required for some or all of the following categories.

1 'Special'

(a) diagnosed blood disease patients

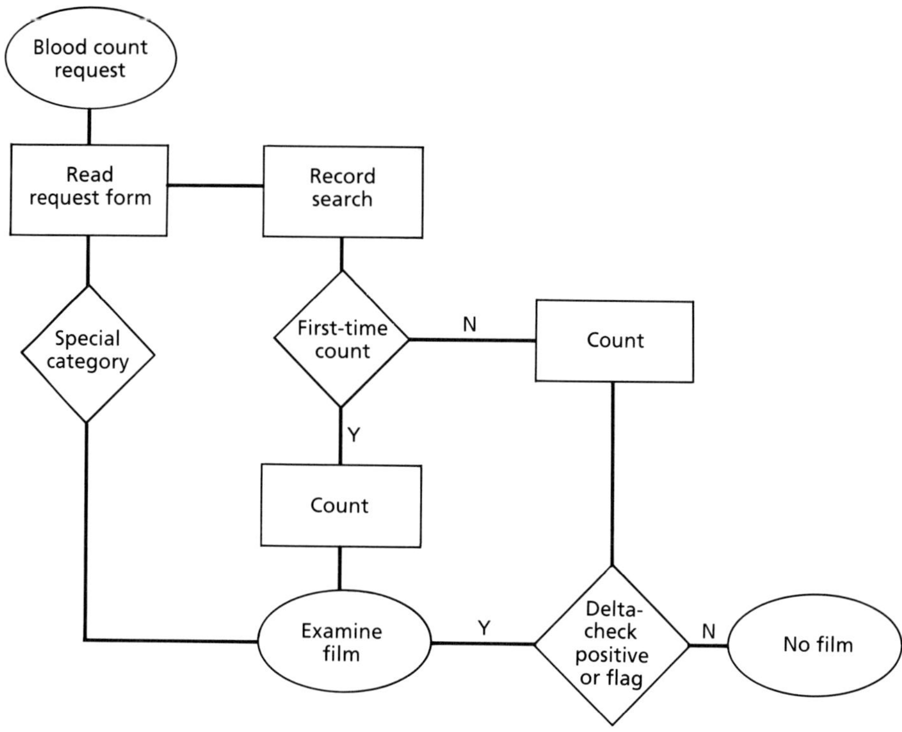

Fig. 4.1 Algorithm for determining the need for blood film examination.

(b) neonates

(c) patients receiving radiotherapy and/or chemotherapy

(d) other patients when indicated by clinical information (e.g. chronic renal failure, infectious mononucleosis).

2 First-time counts.

3 Instrument flag as established for the counter.

4 Significant difference from previous result (delta-check).

For the study, blood specimens were assessed and processed according to normal practice. Blood smears were, however, made from all specimens, whether flagged or not, and examined by a referee. A total of 3500 films were scrutinized in Hospital 2 (Sysmex E5000) and 2400 at Hospital 1 (Coulter S Plus IV). The blood specimens were collected into K_2 EDTA and films were made from these specimens just before the counts were carried out.

Results

In a preliminary trial in Hospital 2, delta-check limits of $\pm 5\%$ for Hb and RBC, $\pm 12\%$ for WBC and platelet count resulted in flagging for film review of over

90% of specimens. When delta-check limits were increased to ± 10% for Hb and RBC, ±20% for WBC and platelets this still resulted in 47% of all subsequent counts being delta-check positive. Accordingly, delta-checking was omitted entirely (Hospital 2) as a result of which, indication for films (for other reasons) was reduced to 70% of cases. On the other hand, at Hospital 1 delta-checking procedure was continued but more realistically at the following limits:

Hb > 2 g/dl < previous result
MCV > 6 fl difference
MCH > 5 pg difference
Normal RDW becoming abnormal
Total WBC normal to abnormal
Clinically inexplicable reduction in platelet count by more than 50%
Changing pattern of histogram.

The distribution of test requests based on the categories defined in the algorithm as described above is given in Table 4.1. The extent of concordance between instrument results and morphological features is shown in Table 4.2.

Table 4.1 Analysis of specimens in survey

	Hospital 2 3500 cases %	Hospital 1 2400 cases %
Film required (Fig. 4.1)	70	61
Clinical indication*	15	11
First time with abnormal count	12	12
Instrument flag	43	28
Delta check	47[†]	30
With other factors	35	20
Only factor	12	10
Film not required	30	39

* Includes all diagnosed blood disorders, neonates, chronic renal failure, radiotherapy and chemotherapy patients.
[†]Not used as indicator for film (see text).

Table 4.2 Concordance between prediction (instrument result) and microscopic scrutiny (referee)

			% Total	
Set	Prediction	Referee	Hospital 2	Hospital 1
True negative (TN)	Normal	Normal	49.6	51.3
True positive (TP)	Abnormal	Abnormal	33.4	36.1
False negative (FN)	Normal	Abnormal	2.7	1.6
False positive (FP)	Abnormal	Normal	14.3	11.0

The terminology used follows that of Galen and Gambino (1975) as applied in the previous chapter. In both centres, in approximately 80–90% of cases, there was good agreement between film and counter, i.e. the film was normal when there had been no indication to scrutinize it and conversely an abnormality was identified when the algorithm had required a film. However, in approximately 15% of cases there was a discrepancy.

Failure of the algorithm was due mainly to the requirement for a film which was subsequently shown to have been unnecessary as no morphological abnormality was seen. The reasons are listed in Table 4.3. Flags with no apparent clinical significance occurred as a result of platelet clumps or fibrin in the samples, in normal neonatal bloods, in chronic renal failure and in blood specimens which had been left for more than 3–4 hours at room temperature before testing. In a significant number of cases, however, no obvious reason for the flagging could be identified on film examination.

The converse reason for failure of the algorithm was a morphological abnormality which was not indicated by the instrument. Those relating to red cells are listed in Table 4.4 and to white cells and other abnormal features in Table 4.5.

The effects of delay in testing beyond 3–4 hours and/or incorrect concentration of EDTA on leucocyte morphology are shown in Table 4.6.

Discussion

In the past two decades there has been a remarkable increase in the numbers of blood counts performed in routine diagnostic laboratories. The advent of automated cell counters marked a major advance, enabling the laboratories to keep pace with this demand except for blood film examination. The blood film has always been an essential component of the 'blood count', for four functions—(i) to perform a full (quantitative) differential leucocyte count, (ii) to obtain a

Table 4.3 False positive instrument flags

	Hospital 2		Hospital 1	
Feature	No.	% cases	No.	% cases
Platelet clumps	53	1.5	34	1.4
Fibrin	28	0.8	22	0.9
EDTA and storage effect	42	1.2	46	1.9
Neonatal	37	1.1	—	—
Unidentified	160	4.6	53	2.2
Chronic renal failure	180	5.1	110	4.6
Total	500	14.3	265	11.0

Table 4.4 Red cell survey*

Abnormalities not flagged by instrument	Film indicated	
	Yes	No
Polychromasia	243	21
Dimorphic	227	22
Target cells	121	11
Spherocytes	44	3
Elliptocytes	10	8
Stomatocytes	1	1
Sickle cells	12	0
Burr cells/schistocytes	142	12
Poikilocytes	31	7
Pencil cells	82	10
Acanthocytes	2	1
Rouleaux	112	28
Autoagglutination	9	11
Howell–Jolly bodies	15	2
Punctate basophilia	9	1
Pappenheimer bodies	2	0

*Data from Hospitals 1 and 2 combined: 5900 specimens

Table 4.5 Leucocyte and other abnormalities*

Feature	Film required	
	Yes†	No
Blast cells	18	7‡
Myelocytes	32	22
Neutrophil left shift	39	10
Hypersegmented neutrophils	44	7
Eosinophilia	16	20
Basophilia	3	4
Reactive lymphocytes	34	18
Atypical mononuclears	16	4
Plasma cells	1	1
Smear cells	5	0
Megakaryocyte fragments	5	0
Nucleated RBC	11	11

*Data from both hospitals combined: 5900 specimens.
†By criteria shown in Fig. 4.1 including instrument flag in some cases.
‡ Not required in these cases as films had been examined and blast cells noted, on previous occasions. No new case of acute leukaemia was missed.

Table 4.6 Effect of storage and EDTA*

Counter	Film	No. of cases
Normal screen	Unsatisfactory	19
Flagged	Satisfactory	43
Flagged	Unsatisfactory	38
Rejected	Satisfactory	36

*Data combined: 5900 specimens.

rough assessment of the leucocyte distribution, (iii) to identify presence of unusual cells such as blasts, myelocytes, nucleated red cells, etc., (iv) to study blood cell morphology.

To examine a film with every count has become impractical and it is necessary to select those films which should be scrutinized and to decide on which of these a full DLC should be undertaken.

The problem of how to select films for scrutiny was studied at Hammersmith Hospital some 24 years ago by Lewis and Hoffbrand (1967). Analysis of the blood counts carried out at that time showed at least one measurement outside the normal reference values in 73% of the specimens, thus making this too sensitive as a criterion. Conversely, in some cases all parameters of the count were within the normal range whereas the blood films showed diagnostic features. However, in most of these cases the need for a film would have been 'flagged' by the clinical presentation. This highlights the importance of providing the laboratory with adequate clinical information to give this criterion a useful role in the selection algorithm.

Since this early study, laboratory practice has undergone major changes in the light of development of automated counting systems. The need for visual DLC has been reduced dramatically by the use of automated counters which provide three-part DLC and even more comprehensively, full five-part DLC by flow cytochemistry, flow cytometry and computerized pattern recognition. There have been a number of reports on evaluations of these systems (e.g. Griswold & Champagne, 1985; Greendyke *et al.*, 1985; Nelson *et al.*, 1985; Pierre *et al.*, 1987; Clarke *et al.*, 1986). These reports have concentrated on comparison of the performance of the counters, comparing automated and manual DLCs. The utility of the former in practice has also been described (Duncan & Gottfried, 1987; Arkin *et al.*, 1987), but specifically with reference to the DLC.

The present study considered all aspects of the blood film and its function in association with the blood count by automated counting systems. In an ideal system flags to indicate the need for a blood film would be sufficiently sensitive and specific to ensure neither missed nor unnecessary film examination. Unfortunately, these requirements tend to be opposing criteria and this study has shown the extent to which each influences the effectiveness of selection of films for scrutiny. Thus, delta-checking resulted in an excessive requirement for films until the limits were greatly widened. Conversely, failure of flagging to alert to an abnormality occurred in a number of cases, as listed in Tables 4.4 and 4.5. The clinical consequence of this is difficult to assess but it is likely that most of these cases would be flagged into one of the 'obligatory film' categories in a subsequent count.

Another aspect of 'flagging' is the marking on the numerical reports of all results which are outside normal reference limits. In the Hospital 2 study these comprised 56% of tests but as many were only at the borderline of abnormal there were no obvious abnormalities in their films. It is, thus, debatable whether the specimens in this group should be included in the 'obligatory film' category.

It must be appreciated that the criteria for film examination described in this chapter reflect the practice in large teaching hospitals with a number of special clinics and with many patients being referred from other regions and other countries for specialist diagnosis and management. Undoubtedly, a greater proportion of films need to be examined under these circumstances than in a district general hospital, as described in Chapter 3. Even so, differences in practice do occur in the former.

Confusion in interpretation and unnecessary flagging may be caused by the effect of incorrect concentration of EDTA and prolonged storage of the specimen before testing. Too little anticoagulant or inadequate mixing of the specimen at the time of collection can result in fibrin formation; excessive anticoagulant affects morphology of the leucocytes and platelets and prolonged storage results in crenation of the red cells and autolysis of leucocytes. Delta-checking may also be affected if there is variable storage of specimens before testing as there is a gradual and progressive increase in MCV and decrease in platelet counts with storage. Platelet counts have shown a decrease of 16% after 12 hours and 34% after 24 hours storage at 4°C although not at room temperature (van Assendelft & Parvin, 1988). The form of EDTA may also affect the MCV and differences of 3% in MCV have been shown between K_2 and K_3 EDTA (van Assendelft & Parvin, 1988). It is thus essential to standardize the specimen collection containers and to set a limit on the time delay between collection and testing. Our personal experience indicates that this should not exceed 3–4 hours.

The efficiency of the automated counters used in this study were assessed by the method of Galen and Gambino (1975), based on the ability of the instrument to identify correctly and specifically abnormalities shown on the film. The results are shown in Table 4.7. The counters have the same degree of efficiency, about 85%. Using the proposed algorithm described above, the blood count data combined with scrutiny of the selected films makes it unlikely that any serious error in blood count performance will occur in the routine laboratory. To achieve

Table 4.7 Efficiency of counters used in survey

	Toa Sysmex E5000 Hospital 2 %	Counter S Plus IV Hospital 1 %	Combined data %
Sensitivity (TP/TP + FN)	93	96	95
Specificity (TN/TN + FP)	80	82	81
Positive predictive value (TP/TP + FP)	70	77	74
Negative predictive value (TN/TN + FN)	95	97	96

TP = true positive, TN = true negative, FP = false positive, FN = false negative.

this in a specialist teaching hospital the system required a film to be examined in approximately 61% of the tests at Hospital 1 and 70% at Hospital 2.

References

Arkin C.F., Medeiros L.J., Pevzner L.Z. *et al.* (1987) The white blood cell differential: evaluation of rapid impression scanning versus the routine manual count. *American Journal of Clinical Pathology* **87**, 628–632.

Clarke A., Garvey B. & Lewis S.M. (1986) *An Evaluation of the Sysmex Toa E5000 Analyzer.* Department of Health and Social Security STB/86/30.

Clarke P.T., Henthorn J.S. & England J.M. (1985) Differential white cell counting on the Coulter Counter Model S Plus IV (three population) and the Technicon H6000; a comparison by simple and multiple regression. *Clinical and Laboratory Haematology* **7**, 335–351.

Duncan K.L. & Gottfried E.L. (1987) Utility of the three part leukocyte differential count. *American Journal of Clinical Pathology* **88**, 308–313.

Galen R.S. & Gambino S.R. (1975) *Beyond normality: The predictive value and efficiency of medical diagnosis.* John Wiley, New York.

Greendyke R.M., Kanter D.R., DeBoover L., Savage L. & Van Gelder S. (1985) A comparison of differential white blood counts using manual, Technicon and Coulter S Plus IV. *American Journal of Clinical Pathology* **84**, 348–350.

Griswold D.J. & Champagne V.D. (1985) Evaluation of the Coulter S Plus IV three-part differential in an acute care hospital. *American Journal of Clinical Pathology* **84**, 49–57.

Lewis S.M. & Hoffbrand A.V. (1967) Automation in perspective. *British Journal of Haematology* **13** (Suppl.) 36–39.

Nelson L., Charache S., Keyser E. & Metzger P. (1985) Laboratory evaluation of the Coulter 'three-part electronic differential'. *American Journal of Clinical Pathology* **83**, 547–554.

Pierre R.V., Payne B.A., Lee W.K. *et al.* (1987) Comparison of four leukocyte differential methods with the National Committee for Clinical Laboratory Standards (NCCLS) Reference Method. *American Journal of Clinical Pathology* **87**, 201–209.

van Assendelft O.W. & Parvin R.M. (1988) Specimen collection, handling and storage. In Lewis S.M. & Verwilghen R.L. (eds) *Quality Assurance in Haematology*, pp. 5–32. Bailliere Tindall, London.

5 Haemoglobinopathy Screening

Prepared by the
General Haematology Task Force

There is an increasing need to screen for sickle haemoglobin (Hb S) in the UK. This chapter provides guidelines on when such screening should be undertaken and on the methods that are recommended. Screening for sickle haemoglobin and thalassaemia is necessary to detect the presence, and when present, to determine the significance of the inherited condition. The application of the guidelines will to some extent depend on the local population structure, but such screening is usually carried out for one or two reasons: (i) to assist in the clinical management of individuals with homozygous conditions and (ii) to provide information for genetic counselling. In these guidelines the term sickle cell disease (SCD) includes the following conditions: homozygous sickle cell anaemia (SS), sickle cell haemoglobin C disease (SC), sickle β^{+}-thalassaemia (Sβ^{+}) and sickle β°-thalassaemia (Sβ°), as well as other rarer combinations such as SD, SE, SO, S hereditary persistence of fetal haemoglobin. The term sickle cell trait is used to describe individuals who are heterozygous for Hb A and Hb S (AS).

Screening for sickle haemoglobin (Hb S)

Screening for Hb S before general anaesthesia

This is required to ensure safety during general anaesthesia, and appropriate postoperative care for individuals with sickle cell trait as well as for those with sickle cell disease (SCD).

Pre-anaesthetic screening should be offered to all patients of African or Afro-Caribbean descent. Whilst the incidence of sickle haemoglobin is also high in some areas of the Middle East, southern Italy, Greece, Turkey, Cyprus and India (Livingstone 1985; Serjeant 1985), in the UK the incidence of sickle haemoglobin in people originating from these countries appears to be low at the time of writing (1987); however, routine screening of these patients before general anaesthesia is also recommended whenever possible. It is important that the

Reprinted with permission from *Clinical and Laboratory Haematology* 1988, **10**, 87–94.

policy be kept under review in the light of changing demographic and immigration patterns, and of the increasing intermarriage between communities.

Antenatal screening

(See also p. 48). Antenatal screening is carried out to detect both SCD and sickle cell trait, thus providing information necessary for the correct management of the pregnancy and also for alerting the clinician to the necessity for screening the father in order to predict the possible risk to the infant. These tests can be undertaken either before or during pregnancy.

Neonatal screening

(See also p. 48). Neonates from *at-risk* communities must be screened at birth for SCD. In the UK, it is expected that at least 1 in 100 African and 1 in 200 Afro-Caribbean babies will be born with SCD. There is a significantly lower mortality and morbidity in infants who are diagnosed at birth and started on prophylactic penicillin by the age of 3 months while at the same time the parents and medical attendants are alerted to the problems to be expected. It is recommended that each region defines its policy for neonatal screening. All mothers at risk should have already been screened for β-thalassaemia trait, sickle haemoglobin and other haemoglobins which interact with β-thalassaemia and/or sickle haemoglobin (see p. 48). It is essential that babies born to mothers carrying these abnormalities, or to mothers who have not previously been tested, are screened at birth. (In order to achieve this it may be necessary in some districts to screen all babies.) Any mothers at risk who have not been tested should also be screened.

Screening for other clinical purposes

The presence of sickle haemoglobin should be excluded in certain clinical conditions known to occur in sickle cell trait and SCD (e.g. haematuria) or in SCD (e.g. aseptic necrosis of hips and shoulders, some types of retinopathy, priapism, etc). Individuals with such conditions should always be screened for the presence of sickle haemoglobin in association with any other investigations undertaken to establish the cause of the problem.

Genetic counselling

All women other than those of Northern European descent should be tested at the antenatal booking clinic for the presence of sickle haemoglobin, other haemoglobin variants and for the β-thalassaemia trait (usually suspected from the characteristic red cell indices obtained on routine blood counts using automated counters). Those found to be heterozygous or homozygous should have their partners tested, so allowing prenatal diagnosis to be offered. Ideally, the tests should be carried out before conception. Screening involves not only the laboratory tests but also counselling and access to antenatal diagnosis. Such a programme should be developed according to the local needs, or the individual should be referred to an appropriate haematological centre.

Testing for sickle haemoglobin

1 The initial routine screen for sickle haemoglobin should always include electrophoresis at alkaline pH (Lehmann & Huntsman, 1966) (usually cellulose acetate), blood film and full blood count with indices. Solubility tests (Lehmann & Huntsman, 1966) should be included.

2 If cellulose acetate electrophoresis shows a band running in the position of haemoglobin S and a sickle solubility test is negative (not applicable to neonates, see 6 below), then citrate agar gel electrophoresis (Lehmann & Huntsman, 1966) should be carried out. This is especially valuable to separate Hb S and Hb D. Citrate agar is also useful in differentiating between Hb C and Hb E.

3 Before reporting the presence of sickle haemoglobin, the haemoglobin concentration and red cell indices (MCV, MCH, or both) should be determined and the blood film examined. Patients referred for sickle screening and found to be negative but to have microcytic, hypochromic red cell indices (Weatherall & Clegg, 1981) should have their Hb A_2 and Hb F levels quantitated and the iron status assessed.

4 If on haemoglobin electrophoresis the proportion of sickle haemoglobin appears to be greater than Hb A, then the quantity of sickle haemoglobin should be determined since such a result may indicate the presence of sickle/β^+-thalassaemia.

5 It is important to know whether or not the individual has been transfused recently since the presence of transfused blood can cause misleading results.

6 Sickle solubility tests (Lehmann & Huntsman, 1966) may produce either false negative or false positive results and should only be used without electrophoresis in cases of emergency (Bates *et al.*, 1985). Negative and positive control samples must always be included and all results should be confirmed by electrophoresis on cellulose acetate at alkaline pH at the earliest opportunity. It is important to remember that the sickle solubility test is of no value in the neonate even when the child has sickle cell anaemia (Hb SS), because it is negative in the presence of a high fetal haemoglobin concentration.

7 Controls: (a) each electrophoretic strip should include control samples containing Hb A, Hb S, and if possible Hb C; (b) a normal blood sample and a sample from a patient with sickle cell trait should be used as negative and positive controls, respectively, each time a sickle solubility test is carried out.

Suggested sickle screening procedure in an emergency

In an emergency there may be insufficient time to wait for the result of electrophoresis and for completion of the screening procedure described above. In this situation the sickle solubility test (see 6 above) and full blood count and indices should be carried out and the peripheral blood film examined. A reticulocyte count is often helpful.

If the sickle solubility test is *negative* no further action is required, but the full screening procedure must be completed at the earliest possible time.

If the sickle solubility test is *positive*, and if the blood count and film are normal, the patient may be presumed to have sickle cell trait, and the local protocol for dealing with anaesthesia in such individuals should be followed.

If the sickle solubility test is *positive*, and the blood film shows sickle or target cells, the patient should be presumed to have SCD irrespective of haemoglobin concentration until proved otherwise as some patients with SCD may have normal haemoglobin concentration. The local arrangements for emergency anaesthesia in SCD must be followed.

On occasion, haemoglobin electrophoresis may be required 'out of hours' but it should only be undertaken after consultation with a consultant haematologist. In centres which carry out paediatric surgery, emergency haemoglobin electrophoresis should be carried out because the sickle solubility test may remain negative for the first few months of life in babies with sickle cell trait as well as those with SCD. (This is in part due to the variable sensitivity of different solubility reagents that are available on the market (Weatherhall & Clegg, 1981).) The problem could be avoided if all at-risk babies were screened at birth and their genotype established, properly recorded and available to the clinician.

In order to ensure adequate anaesthetic management of those with sickle cell trait and of patients with SCD, the screening for sickle haemoglobin should only be carried out in departments supervised by a consultant haematologist and participating in the National External Quality Assessment Scheme. Participation in a local quality assurance scheme is also desirable.

Information about the results of screening

Each individual tested should be informed of the result. A card giving the haemoglobin genotype should be available nationally, preferably published by the

DoH in a similar fashion to the transplant card (for suggested design see Fig. 5.1). An explanatory leaflet on sickle haemoglobin which includes the details of local

(a)

Front	Back
UK HAEMOGLOBINOPATHY CARD Mr/Mrs/Miss .... Address .... D.O.B. .... Hospital No. .... Has been tested and found to have: Date tested .... Signed .... Hospital	LABORATORY RESULTS Date tested: .... Hb Electrophoresis .... Hb F .... % Typical blood count: Hb .... g/dl Retics.............. % This inherited condition may be associated with episodes of pain, infection or profound anaemia. Should there be any queries concerning this patient, please contact the address given on the front of this card.

(b)

Front	Back
UK HAEMOGLOBINOPATHY CARD Mr/Mrs/Miss .... Address .... D.O.B. .... Hospital No. .... Has been tested and found to have: Date tested .... Signed .... Hospital	LABORATORY RESULTS Date tested: .... Hb Electrophoresis .... Hb A_2 .... %, Hb F.............. % Typical blood count: Hb .... g/dl Retics.............. % Should there be any queries concerning this patient, please contact the address given on the front of this card.

(c)

Front	Back
UK HAEMOGLOBINOPATHY CARD Mr/Mrs/Miss .... Address .... D.O.B. .... has the inherited condition Date tested .... Signed .... Hospital	**This inherited condition is NOT a disease. If further details are required they can be obtained from a Sickle Cell/Thalassaemia Information Centre, or from the address given on the front of this card.**

(d)

Front	Back
UK HAEMOGLOBINOPATHY CARD Mr/Mrs/Miss .... Address .... D.O.B. .... Has been tested and found to have no evidence of Sickle cell haemoglobin or β-thalassaemia trait. Date tested .... Signed .... Hospital	

Fig. 5.1 Haemoglobinopathy cards. We suggest that the cards of the following type are given to the people who have been tested. They should be designed to fit inside a plastic envelope, the same size as a credit card. (a) Sickle cell disease; (b) other haemoglobinopathies; (c) carrier states; (d) normals.

services should also be available. In addition, the requesting doctor and, in the case of self referral, the patient's general practitioner, should be informed of the result of the sickle screening. Patients found to have one of the varieties of SCD should be referred to a consultant haematologist.

Individuals in need of genetic counselling or who have requested further information should be referred for detailed counselling and information. A mechanism for registering individuals with SCD must be established for each region or district to enable the collection of appropriate statistical data.

Antenatal haemoglobinopathy screening

Objectives

To identify couples at risk of having a child with Hb Barts hydrops fetalis, β-thalassaemia major or sickle cell disease (SS, SC, SD, SE, $S\beta^{\circ}$-thal, $S\beta^{+}$-thal) in time to allow second trimester prenatal diagnosis where appropriate. The tests should be completed by 16 weeks although in exceptional circumstances completion may be deferred to 20 weeks. As first trimester diagnosis is now available it is preferable to screen and counsel the couples before pregnancy, or early enough in pregnancy to allow first trimester diagnosis to be carried out.

The following are basic recommendations.

1 (a) All women should be screened at booking for thalassaemia by measurement of red cell indices. If MCV < 76 fl and/or the MCH < 27 pg* then the Hb A_2 and F should be quantitated and the iron status assessed†. (b) All women except those of Northern European extraction should be screened by haemoglobin electrophoresis for the presence of sickle haemoglobin, or an abnormal haemoglobin which interacts with sickle haemoglobin.

2 If any of the women tested in **1** (a) or (b) is diagnosed as having AS, AC, AD, AE, β-thalassaemia trait, Hb Lepore or SS, SC, SD, SE, $S\beta^{\circ}$-thal, $S\beta^{+}$-thal, then the father should be tested using tests in **1** (a) and (b) above. Ideally the father should also be tested if the woman is microcytic regardless of her Hb A_2 concentration. (a) If the father is normal, no further action is required. (b) If the father is heterozygous or homozygous for a haemoglobin abnormality then the couple should be referred without delay to a specialist centre for counselling and for consideration of prenatal diagnosis when required. (c) If the pregnant woman

* Different laboratories using different types of cell counter may use different values for the indices, e.g. MVC < 80 fl and MCH < 29 pg. The MCH may be a better guide than the MCV when using some automated cell counters.

† At the present time (1986) it is not feasible to screen *reliably and routinely* for α-thalassaemia trait. Globin chain synthesis and gene mapping can be arranged for couples at risk of having a baby with thalassaemia major (Hb Barts hydrops fetalis).

has β-thalassaemia trait, Hb Lepore trait, sickle cell trait or Hb E trait and if the father's blood picture is microcytic, but he is not iron deficient and has a normal Hb A_2 with no evidence of α-thalassaemia trait (such as Hb H bodies) then ideally the couple should be referred for globin chain synthesis studies to exclude β-thalassaemia trait with a normal Hb A_2. (d) If the father is unavailable for testing, whenever possible the mother should be counselled.

Neonatal haemoglobinopathy screening

Objectives

To detect babies with $\beta°$-thalassaemia major or sickle cell disease (SS, SC, SD, SE, $S\beta°$-thalassaemia). Unfortunately $S\beta^+$-thalassaemia* and β^+-thalassaemia major cannot always be reliably detected at or soon after birth by the methods outlined below.

The following are basic recommendations (International Committee for Standardization in Haematology 1988):

1 Test cord blood or a heel prick sample from all babies at risk, i.e. babies of mothers with AS, AC, AD, AE, SS, SC, SD, SE, $S\beta^+$-thal, $S\beta^+$-thal or β-thalassaemia trait. However, in some districts to achieve this it may be necessary to test all newborn babies. Cord blood specimens must be collected by venepuncture of the umbilical vein to avoid contamination with maternal blood.†

2 Each blood sample should be examined electrophoretically using a technique which gives good separation of Hb A and Hb F, i.e. on cellulose acetate at alkaline pH as recommended by the ICSH. If any abnormality is detected, citrate agar gel electrophoresis at acid pH should also be undertaken.

3 Babies provisionally diagnosed as having SS, SC, SD, SE, $S\beta$-thalassaemia or β-thalassaemia major should be retested not later than at 3 months and if the diagnosis is confirmed, they should be followed in a paediatric haematology clinic so that they can be appropriately managed and treated from an early age.

* Ideally AS babies should be retested between the ages of 4 and 6 months to exclude $S\beta^+$-thalassaemia but this may not be feasible at the present time.

† Cord blood samples may sometimes be contaminated with maternal blood. It is very important that any such contamination is detected since even a small amount of adult contamination will make Hb F + S (probable sickle cell anaemia) look like Hb F + A + S (sickle cell trait). Such contamination may result in the Hb A band being stronger than the Hb F band or an Hb F + A pattern having the appearance of an Hb F + A + C pattern due to the presence of Hb A_2. If a cord blood sample gives such an appearance a blood film should be made and a cytochemical test for Hb F, such as the Kleihauer test, carried out. Unless maternal contamination can be excluded by this means a fresh specimen should be obtained from the baby and tested. If blood is obtained from the cut end of the cord, up to 20% of samples may be contaminated with maternal blood but if the specimen is obtained by venepuncture of an umbilical vein such contamination is much less likely. If possible the tests should be repeated on a fresh specimen whenever an abnormality is detected since this will reduce errors resulting from contamination with maternal blood.

Acknowledgements

A.J. Bellingham and the late G.W. Marsh participated in the preparation of these guidelines and their help is gratefully acknowledged.

Appendix: Report on JOSHUA

An evaluation of the JOSHUA sickle screening kit was completed at the Central Middlesex Hospital in the summer of 1989. This kit uses a monoclonal antibody and a colour change to detect the presence of haemoglobin S. A protocol for testing was devised to establish the reliability of the JOSHUA test in emergency screening for Hb S, its suitability for testing neonatal and infant blood samples, and the kit stability.

The kit proved to be reliable in detecting Hb S in liquid adult, and baby blood samples provided the concentration of the Hb S was at least 0.5 g/dl in the sample tested. Liquid blood samples collected into the anticoagulant and treated according to the manufacturer's instructions remained stable and showed clear positive results even after 4 weeks of storage. Six hundred neonatal samples collected directly onto filter paper were also tested; JOSHUA detected Hb S reliably and consistently. The original lot of kits (all of the same batch number) submitted for testing gave rise to a small number of false positive results. The fault was due to a defective urease reagent. The subsequent batches tested did not have this fault and proved reliable when used in a variety of situations.

JOSHUA is a quick and reliable screening test for Hb S. Like the solubility and sickling tests it cannot distinguish between the heterozygote and the homozygote state. Its main advantage is its ability reliably to detect Hb S in the presence of even large proportions of Hb F in both liquid and filter paper samples of blood. It is a costly test (the cost per test including technical time varies between £3.00 and £7.00 depending on whether a single test or a batch of tests is performed). Nevertheless there is a definitive place for the JOSHUA test in paediatric emergencies and for confirming the presence of Hb S in the neonatal screening programmes, provided the manufacturer ensures that the reagents in each batch of kits are stringently checked.

References

Association of Clinical Pathologists (1975) Laboratory detection of haemoglobinopathies. *Broadsheet* **33**.

Bates, J., Edwards N., Hyde K., Burgess R., Hunt L.P., Lenerhan H. & MacIver J.E. (1985) *An evaluation of sickle haemoglobin (Hb S) screening methods.* DHSS, Scientific and Technical Branch, Report No. STB 3A/85/41. Obtainable from Mr Kennedy (Tel. 071 636 6811, ex. 3377).

International Committee for Standardization in Haematology (1988) *Recommended method for neonatal haemoglobinopathy screening.* In press.

Lehmann H. & Huntsman R.G. (1966) *Man's Haemoglobins*, pp. 262–298. North-Holland Publishing Company, Amsterdam.

Livingstone F.B. (1985) *Frequencies of Hemoglobin Variants.* Oxford University Press, New York.

Serjeant G.R. (1985) *Sickle Cell Disease*, pp. 18–23. Oxford University Press, Oxford.

Serjeant G.R. (1985) *Sickle Cell Disease*, pp. 18–23. Oxford University Press, Oxford.

Weatherall D.J. & Clegg J.B. (1981) *The Thalassaemia Syndromes*, 3rd edn, pp. 222–227. Blackwell Scientific Publications, Oxford.

6 Computing for General Haematology

Prepared by the General Haematology Task Force

Introduction

Computer systems have become essential since manual data processing cannot cope with constantly increasing numbers of requests, and tests per request. A computer is capable of manipulating large quantities of data automatically. The resulting benefits include the following points.

1 Improved speed and accuracy of data handling:

(a) on-line links for instruments,

(b) mechanisms to reduce clerical transcription errors at the input stage,

(c) error trapping procedures,

(d) improved quality control, and

(e) facilitation of calculations.

2 Improved methods of data retrieval permitting quick response to enquiry. With manual methods it is often difficult to locate work in progress or results which are waiting to be filed or which are misfiled.

3 Compilation of up-to-date and accurate information, less readily available from manual systems, required for workload returns and for budgeting, planning and research purposes.

Laboratory computer systems must be sufficiently flexible that they do not impose their own rigid work pattern on the laboratory and they must also be able to cope with multiple users and with fluctuations in demand during the working day without response times being degraded. It is essential that the system continues to function, albeit more slowly, in the event of major component failure. To achieve this objective it is helpful to have major items of equipment linked to microcomputers.

Consideration should be given to the integration of the computer system for haematology and blood transfusion because of their clinical interdependence in the hospital setting.

Links with other pathology disciplines are important for the transfer of data but shared computing facilities may not be sufficiently flexible and may result in slow response times. Compatibility with other computer systems in the hospital is important since this allows efficient links, at reasonable cost, to clinical and administrative areas.

It is not, of course, possible to write a generalized specification for a haematology computer system. Since laboratories vary both in workload and in type of work, they will be equipped and operate in different ways. They also have individual problems in how to distribute results to the various hospitals and clinics that they serve but these may be minimized if a hospital information system exists. Nevertheless, it is hoped that the guidelines given below will be helpful when operational requirements are drawn up for individual departments.

Data input

Patient details

DEMOGRAPHY

The most important area to consider is the input of patient identification data. As a minimum there should be a unique patient number, surname, forename(s), sex, date of birth (if possible rather than age), together with the name of the requesting consultant or GP and the source, for example ward name, clinic, etc.

Sites with a master patient index system (MPI) must include in any specification a requirement that the proposed computer system has facilities for accessing the MPI for patient demographic data.

If the hospital does not have a master index, then it is necessary for an index to be built up on the haematology system. This index can then be interrogated by giving an abbreviated identity, for example identification number and surname. If the full identity conforms with that on the request then it is not necessary to input the remaining details of identity. When such an index is not available each identification will have to be entered in full at a VDU. Data entered in this way for any patient is likely to differ slightly from request to request, for example by giving an age or a date of birth, so that the possibilities for cumulative reporting will be reduced. This difficulty can be circumvented if a 'merging' routine is available for use by sufficiently experienced staff.

In some hospitals the patient details and tests requested may be directly entered in the ward or outpatient clinic via VDUs.

CLINICAL DETAILS

It is desirable to have a facility for entry of limited clinical details including ethnic origin where appropriate.

OTHER DETAILS

The date and time of input should be recorded; this will generally be done automatically by the system.

Special flag codes which enable patients or requests to be identified by specific criteria should be input at this stage, for example high risk, private patient, out-of-hours, drug trials.

Flags may be permanent for all entries on certain patients (e.g. high risk) or be variable (e.g. out-of-hours).

Tests requested

Unless the tests have been requested at a remote terminal, the details of the request will have to be entered at a VDU in the laboratory. The computer system should be capable of operating without worklists, for example for full blood counts. However, this facility should be available if required, for example for serum B12 assays, because batches of samples are accumulated over an interval of several days.

Specimen identification number

Test requests and results need to be uniquely identified and linked to the patient demographic data. This is best achieved by means of specimen identification numbers. If these numbers are not input by an automated device, for example bar code reader, manual entries must include a check character.

Result input

RESULTS FROM AUTOMATED EQUIPMENT

Blood count results and any other results obtained on automated instruments should pass directly 'on-line' to a computer. This could be a dedicated microcomputer with an ability to hold at least 1 day's results in the event of failure of the main haematology computer. At intervals during the working day data should be down-loaded from the microcomputer to the main haematology computer.

Some instruments have a data storage capacity available either routinely or as an optional extra; however this is mainly for internal quality control purposes and may not be sufficient to store 1 day's workload.

RESULTS OBTAINED MANUALLY

These results are normally entered via a VDU. Mechanisms to avoid or reduce transcription errors are advantageous, for example comparison of results entered independently on two occasions.

DIFFERENTIAL WHITE CELL COUNT AND BLOOD FILM REPORT

When a VDU is used for differential counting the keys should be designated so that they can be pressed for each cell type and an audible signal given when the predetermined number of cells have been differentiated. The number of cells to be counted should be variable and the number of cell types within the differential should be consistent with easy manipulation of the keyboard. The total and differential leucocyte count will require correction for the number of nucleated red cells present.

Commonly used comments on film appearances may be coded but the number should be kept to a minimum for easy memorization. Such comments should include both descriptive terms and actions advised. A facility should also be provided for brief free-text entry. Previous results should be readily available on the same VDU screens while reporting a blood film.

TEXT

The system must support coded comment entry and free text entry with word processing capabilities for reports of marrow morphology, histology, cytochemistry, etc.

URGENT RESULTS

The computer system must be sufficiently flexible to allow the processing of urgent specimens by interrupting batched operations.

Calculation of derived results

Facilities for generating purely mathematical results, for example absolute differential counts, absolute reticulocyte counts and red cell folates should be included.

Quality control, editing and authorization

Quality control

The system should allow whatever quality control procedures are required by the user, for example Shewhart charts and CUSUMs for results from control materials, moving averages of patients' results, delta-checks (difference between the latest result and the previous values from that patient), etc.

It is also useful to check for any data corruption or transcription errors by error trapping checks; these ensure that variables which are related to each other do so correctly, for example calculation of red cell indices from RBC, Hb and PCV, summation of differential percentage values to 100. Checks should also be made for extreme values incompatible with life, for example Hb = 0.1 g/dl or for such grossly unusual values that might merit confirmation by re-analysis, for example Hb = 3.0 g/dl, just to ensure that there has been no unlikely error.

With automated equipment some of these procedures may be performed on computing facilities supplied as part of the instrument package, on the dedicated microcomputer or on the main haematology computer. When designing the system it may be wise to minimize dependence on computing facilities supplied by the instrument manufacturers since future replacement of the instrument will cause less difficulty.

Edit facilities

These are required to enable authorized personnel to correct errors recognized by quality control checks.

Authorization

Once quality control checks have been accomplished and editing performed, results can be authorized. Authorization is carried out by a person of appropriate seniority for the particular type of test which has been performed. Direct authorization may be performed at a work station by the operator. Alternatively, authorization may be performed at a remote VDU screen; this may be of individual or listed results. Although time-consuming the call-up of previous results helps validation. Whichever method is selected, the system should record who has authorized the results.

Reporting

Individual patients

SINGLE REPORTS

The system should allow as many options as possible as requirements differ between requesting departments and hospitals. Either full printed reports should be produced or labels which can be attached to the request. This second option allows the requesting doctor to see the clinical details on the form he/she originally completed, a feature which is often helpful when clinicians are reviewing large numbers of results obtained on outpatients seen over the last few days. However, this requires manual sorting and is time-consuming.

CUMULATIVE REPORTS

In some instances cumulative reports may be helpful. These can only be meaningful if particular care is taken to ensure that each request is accompanied by a full and accurate set of demographic details for the patient. No system should make cumulative reporting mandatory since this can impose heavy overheads and cause significant delays.

For haematology patients it is desirable to present cumulative reports in a graphical form integrating both the general haematology chart and details of blood transfusion support.

INTERIM REPORTS

The facility to issue incomplete reports, for example blood count without differential or ESR, permits early issue of more urgent results.

REPORT FORMAT

The format for printed results must be sufficiently flexible to satisfy the user's requirements. In general it is better for results to be put onto pre-printed stationery (or labels) since this allows reference ranges to be printed clearly, in small type if need be. Units can also be pre-printed, for example $\times 10^9/1$, since such units tend not to be reproduced very well by rapid computer printers and they have to be expressed in a way which may not be readily understood, for example E9/1.

REPORT PRINTING

Results may be printed either as they arise or in larger batches. Larger batches can be sorted by ward but a high-speed printer may be required.

Combined reports and/or searches on more than one patient

It may be helpful to produce combined reports for certain wards, clinics or consultants, for example for case review conferences. The medical staff in the laboratory may also find it helpful to list out all patients with certain haematological abnormalities, for example macrocytosis or thrombocytopenia.

It is with such specialized combined reports that cumulative reporting may be most helpful, allowing the clinician to identify trends and the haematology staff to see what work has been done already, or is in hand, on patients with haematological abnormalities.

Outstanding work list

This provides a list or account of patients and specimens from the work file. Such a list can be of completed but not authorized work, incomplete work or both. The ability to generate an outstanding work list is a useful management tool.

Enquiries

For users within the laboratory there should be free exchange of information between the general haematology and the transfusion systems as well as with any other pathology computers.

Results should only be available for telephone enquiries or visible on remote VDUs if the appropriate quality control procedures are satisfactory. Depending on the organization of the laboratory it may be decided to make only authorized results available in this way.

Ideally remote VDUs should be linked to a hospital information system as well as to the haematology computer. A hospital information system is a computer undertaking the communication function. With such a configuration the haematology computer and the computer holding the patient master index would be linked to the information system as would be the remote VDUs. Enquiries would be drawn from the haematology computer by the information system. Similarly the haematology computer might interrogate the MPI via the information system.

If remote VDUs are used for enquiries appropriate security procedures will need to be installed.

Workload statistics

The DoH already require statistics compiled in a specific way and the system must provide this information. It is likely that more sophisticated measures of workload will be required both to assess efficiency and to assist with clinical budgeting. Thought should be given to how these requirements might be implemented.

Storage of results

On-line

All results for the previous 12 months must be stored on-line. Some results must be stored for longer periods, or indefinitely if certain criteria are met, for example haematological case still alive and under follow-up.

Off-line

Earlier results may be stored off-line either on disc or tape. It is a convenient safeguard against computer failure to have hard-copy print-out. Such copies may be essential if the computer system does not run fulltime. One suitable approach is to produce daily and monthly lists of results arranged in alphabetical order. The daily lists can be discarded when the relevant month's list has been produced. The monthly lists do not usually cause any storage problem but if need be they can be microfilmed or produced directly onto microfiche.

Back-up copies

It is essential to have back-up copies of all programs held on the computer. Copies of patient data should be made at least once a day.

Security

The Data Protection Act (1984) restricts access to data held on computers and these requirements must be observed.

Authorization of reports, 'merging' of patient identification and alteration of any data must only be undertaken by users who satisfy appropriate security checks. Security checks are also necessary at remote VDUs.

Installation, servicing and training

Some requirements may be needed for humidity control, temperature control and electrical supply.

The service contract must stipulate an adequate engineer response time.

It may be desirable for senior haematology staff to be trained in depth at the supplier's education facility. Those who use the computer on a more routine basis can then be trained on site.

Acknowledgements

This chapter has drawn heavily on discussions held by the Haematology Sub-committee, Northwest Thames Regional Health Authority and the document produced for the Sub-committee by Dr S. Ardeman and Mr R. Sale, Edgware General Hospital. Mr D.I. Fish assisted in the preparation of the final draft.

Appendix: A note on the use of computers in clinical haematology

Prepared by the Clinical Haematology Task Force

The management of all patients receiving continuous care in haematology departments may be improved by the use of computers which are especially useful where patients are likely to be in the care of the department for long periods.

To facilitate the storage and reproduction of basic haematological data, links should be established with the basic laboratory computer and, when purchasing computer hardware, it is important to ensure compatibility.

The reproduction of material in the form of a graphical display or chart is important to most groups of haematology patients and special care is needed to ensure not only that newly purchased computers can provide such displays, but also that the graphics are adaptable to the increasing complexity of laboratory and patient data.

Storage and access to protocols in use

Examples of clinical usage in disease states in which data may be most appropriately stored on a computer include: (i) haemoglobinopathies including sickle cell disease; (ii) haematological malignancies; (iii) haemophilia and related coagulation disorders; and (iv) anticoagulant therapy. Specific examples of the use of computers might include the following.

HAEMOPHILIA

The identification of batches of factor VIII used in patient treatment. Notification of the sites and frequency of clinical bleeding.

HAEMATOLOGICAL MALIGNANCIES

Monitoring of drug treatment; transfusion of blood products. Reproduction of patient charts, including blood counts, episodes of bleeding and infection.

ANTICOAGULANT CLINICS

As a data base for diagnosis and anticoagulant dosage. Clinic management (attendance lists).

7 The Assessment of Glucose-6-Phosphate Dehydrogenase Deficiency

Prepared by the General Haematology Task Force

Introduction

Glucose-6-phosphate dehydrogenase (G6PD) is the red cell enzyme which is essential for the production of the NADPH which is needed to keep the glutathione in the reduced state (GSH). Failure of this process will impair the ability of the red cell to deal with oxidative stresses which in turn can lead to haemolytic episodes and anaemia which may be very severe and in some cases fatal.

At least 300 million people are affected by G6PD deficiency. A large number of variants (more than 300) have been described and these may differ in their physiological activity and/or other biochemical properties. The most common of these variants are found in people who originated from the Mediterranean countries (the Mediterranean type), parts of Africa (the African type) and parts of India and South East Asia (Beutler, 1971; Dacie, 1985; Grimes, 1980; Wintrobe, 1981). The geographical areas affected are those where malaria was and may still be prevalent and for this reason G6PD deficiency may coexist in a patient who also has thalassaemia and/or sickle cell disease, as these conditions also occur in people who originate from similar parts of the world.

Some antimalarial drugs can cause oxidative stress to the red cell and therefore it is important to test patients for G6PD deficiency before starting some antimalarial therapy. Although many drugs have been claimed to cause haemolysis in G6PD deficiency, only a few have been well documented to be causative agents (Table 7.1). Bacterial and viral infections are important causes of haemolysis in patients with G6PD deficiency. G6PD deficiency should also be considered in many other clinical situations as described in Table 7.2.

The severity and course of a haemolytic episode depends both on the type of G6PD variant of the patient and the type of oxidative stress. Haemolysis is usually milder with the African type of variant than with the Mediterranean type.

The gene controlling the production of G6PD is located on the X chromosome. Males are therefore hemizygotes, whereas females may be either homozygotes or heterozygotes and a heterozygous female will be a mosaic for the normal and a deficient G6PD enzyme. This variable mixture of normal and deficient red cells makes the diagnosis in some female heterozygotes difficult, especially when using screening tests. Such individuals are usually less severely affected than homozygous females or hemizygous males.

Table 7.1 Drugs and chemicals associated with significant haemolysis in subjects with G6PD deficiency (see Luzzato & Mehta, 1989)

Drugs	Definite association	Possible association
Antimalarials	Primaquine, pamaquine	Chloroquine
Sulphonamides	Pentaquine Sulphanilamide Sulphacetamide Sulphapyridine Sulphamethoxazole	 Sulphamethoxypyridazine Sulphadimidine
Sulphones	Thiazolesulfone Diaminodiaphenylsulphone (DDS, dapsone)	
Nitrofurane	Nitrofurantoin	
Antipyretic-analgesic	Acetanilid	
Others	Nalidixic acid Naphthalene Niridazole Phenylhydrazine Toluidine blue Trinitrotoluene (TNT) Methylene blue Phenazopyridine	Chloramphenicol Vitamin K analogues

Table 7.2 Indications for G6PD testing

Prior to treatment with certain antimalarial drugs (see Table 7.1)
Haemolytic disease of the newborn (non-immune)
Haemolysis associated with 'oxidant' drugs (see Table 7.1)
Red cell morphology suggestive of oxidant damage
Unexplained haemolytic anaemia
Favism
Haemoglobinuria
Sickle cell disease, because sickle cell disease and G6PD deficiency may both occur in the same individual
Family history of G6PD deficiency or favism

Principles of measurement of G6PD activity

G6PD promotes the conversion of its specific substrate glucose-6-phosphate (G6P) to 6-phosphogluconate (6PG) with a simultaneous reduction of the coenzyme NADP to NADPH. The 6PG produced is the substrate for the next enzyme in the metabolic pathway, 6-phosphogluconate dehydrogenase (6PGD), which is also present in the red cells, and which also reduces an additional amount of NADP to NADPH. Since NADPH is produced by both reactions the only way that the true G6PD activity can be measured is by carrying out assays with two different reaction mixtures: one containing an excess of both G6P and 6PG and the other containing only 6PG. The difference in activity between the first (G6PD + 6PGD) and the second (6PGD) assay gives the true G6PD activity (Glock & McLean, 1953). However, for most clinical purposes the WHO (1967) method which measures the overall reaction is quite satisfactory and is simpler to carry out as it only requires two reaction cuvettes whereas the Glock and McLean method requires four reaction cuvettes. All tests for measuring G6PD activity depend on detecting the rate of reduction of NADP to NADPH and are based on one of the following properties of NADPH.

1 Absorption of light at 340 nm.
2 Fluorescence produced by long wavelength UV light (approximately 340 nm).
3 Ability to decolorize or lead to the precipitation of certain dyes.

Factors affecting clinical interpretation

With some G6PD variants, including the African type, young red cells and particularly reticulocytes contain much higher levels of G6PD activity than mature red cells. For this reason tests carried out during, or soon after, a haemolytic episode may give misleading results and in such cases the test should be repeated several months after the haemolytic episode is over. If it is important to make a diagnosis without waiting several months it is possible to make 'correction' for the presence of young red cells and reticulocytes (Herz *et al.*, 1970). Alternatively since the activity of some other red cell enzymes is similarly affected by age a knowledge of their activity can be used for this purpose and this approach will also take into account the effect of any older cells lost by haemolysis. Both hexokinase and 6-phosphogluconate dehydrogenase (6PGD) have been used for this purpose but 6PGD is the most convenient since it has to be assayed as part of the Glock and McLean procedure (see Appendix), which is the basis of the ICSH recommended method (ICSH, 1977).

Neither of the screening tests has an unequivocal end-point and this makes interpretation difficult with some samples. If a group of normal samples (say 20) are tested, it will help the analyst recognize the appropriate end-point. Ideally a mixture of normal and deficient red cells should be prepared so as to produce a sample with approximately 50% of the mean 'normal' activity. This sample should then be used to establish an appropriate end-point for the screening tests.

Screening tests (fluorescence or dye decolorization) are useful to differentiate between normal and grossly deficient samples, but neither of these techniques can reliably detect G6PD deficiency in heterozygote women. Equivocal results are difficult to interpret. It is advisable that the activity of these as well as of all deficient samples be confirmed by quantitative assay if at all possible.

Anaemic samples and samples with a high leucocyte count can give misleading results in both the fluorescent and decolorization screening tests. These problems can be avoided if the buffy coat is removed and packed red cells are used instead of whole blood in these screening tests.

Specimen collection and storage

For quantitative assays and for the fluorescence screening test normal blood samples anticoagulated with EDTA, heparin or ACD can be stored for up to 3 weeks at 4°C or up to 5 days at room temperature with less than 10% loss of G6PD activity (Beutler, 1984). Samples containing variants may be less stable than samples containing the normal enzyme. However a fresh sample (less than 24 hours old) is required for dye decolorization tests and heparin should not be used as an anticoagulant for these tests as it may affect the decolorization time. The cytochemical test must be carried out on the day of the blood collection if anticoagulated with EDTA or heparin or within 1 week if ACD is used. Since G6PD in haemolysates is unstable at room temperature, 4°C or −20°C, haemolysates should not be stored. In summary we recommend that whole blood samples be stored for not more than 5 days if anticoagulated with EDTA or for not more than 3 weeks if anticoagulated with ACD.

Laboratory methods

If a man or woman is suspected of having G6PD deficiency on clinical grounds they should be investigated initially by either the fluorescent or the dye decolorization screening test. If the screening test is abnormal or borderline the quantitative assay should be undertaken to confirm, or refute, the diagnosis. If a woman has an equivocal result in the quantitative assay then the cytochemical assay should be undertaken. If there is a clinical or genetic reason to suspect that a woman is heterozygous for G6PD deficiency then the cytochemical assay should be undertaken even if the quantitative assay is normal because as stated below, the cytochemical assay may be the only way to detect a deficiency in some heterozygote women. After a haemolytic episode all the tests may give normal or borderline results even though the individual has G6PD deficiency. For this reason it is sometimes essential to retest a patient 4 months or more after a haemolytic episode in order to ensure that the diagnosis of G6PD deficiency is not missed. In the clinical situation the WHO quantitative technique is satisfactory but has the disadvantage that the activity of 6-phosphogluconate dehydrogenase is not measured and therefore cannot be used to assess the effect of young red cells and reticulocytes. After a haemolytic episode or if the reticulocyte count is raised the Glock and McLean (1953) technique gives more information and this will assist with the interpretation.

If G6PD deficiency is confirmed the implications should be explained to the patient who should also be given a 'card' containing the relevant information. A suggested format for such a card is given in Figure 7.1.

The following is a brief description of various laboratory tests which may be used for the diagnosis of G6PD deficiency together with practical points which may be useful to the analyst. Laboratories undertaking these screening tests and assays should participate in National and Regional Quality Assurance Schemes.

Fluorescent screening test

A procedure based on the method recommended by the ICSH (1979) is given in the Appendix to this chapter. Blood is mixed with an appropriate reaction mixture containing a detergent to lyse the red cells. After a standard time the

This card should be shown to the doctor if you need medical treatment.

Name ____________

The bearer of this card has

A DEFICIENCY OF RED CELL G6PD*

(Glucose 6 phosphate dehydrogenase)

Issued by:
Doctor's Signature ____________

Date ____________

In case of difficulty contact:

Doctor ____________

____

____

Telephone ____________

* see over for further details.

Glucose 6 phosphate dehydrogenase deficiency

Enzyme level ____________ Normal range ____________

Some of the common drugs and chemicals which may cause haemolysis of the red cells in patients with G6PD deficiency are listed below:

Acetanilide	Phenazopyridine
Chloramphenicol	Phenylhydrazine
Dapsone	Sulphacetamide
Methylene blue	Sulphadimidine
Nalidixic acid	Sulphamethoxazole
Naphthalene	Sulphanilamide
Nitrofurantoin and allied drugs	Sulphapyridine
Pamaquine	Toluidine blue
Pentaquine	Trinitrotoluene (TNT)
	Vitamin K

Fig. 7.1 Card to be carried by a patient with G6PD deficiency.

mixture is 'spotted' onto filter paper, dried and inspected under long wavelength UV light. The appearance and brightness of the fluorescence due to NADPH gives a measure of the activity of G6PD.

Dye decolorization screening test

A freshly prepared haemolysate is added to the reaction mixture containing a coloured dye at an appropriate concentration. The rate of decolorization of the dye by the NADPH produced gives a measure of the activity of G6PD. In the Motulsky Test (Motulsky *et al.*, 1959) described in the Appendix the dye is brilliant cresyl blue, while in the Sigma colorimetric test (Procedure No. 400) 2, 6-dichlorophenol indophenol is used. Unfortunately only certain batches of brilliant cresyl blue are suitable for the dye decolorization test and so it is important that all new batches are tested for suitability.

Reagent kits for both the fluorescent test and the dye decolorization test can be obtained commercially and the Sigma Kits have been assessed by Lewis and Saunders (1989).

Cytochemical assay

The technique described by Fairbanks and Lampe (1968) is satisfactory and is summarized in the Appendix. It is based on the fact that haemoglobin can reduce certain dyes to form a granular precipitate while methaemoglobin (MetHb) cannot do this. The test involves a preliminary incubation of red cells with nitrite to change all the haemoglobin to methaemoglobin. This is followed by a second incubation with a reaction mixture containing the dye. The presence of G6PD in the red cells leads to the formation of NADPH which reduces methaemoglobin to haemoglobin and hence precipitation of the dye to form granules. The presence of these granules in the red cells therefore indicates G6PD activity. Counting the granules in the red cells can give a semi-quantitative assessment of G6PD. This method may sometimes be the only way to identify G6PD deficiency in some heterozygous females. However in some women the effects of Lyonization of the X-chromosome are such that even this test may fail to detect the heterozygous state and in such cases the only way to diagnose the condition is by family studies or by DNA analysis. However DNA analysis is only practical if the precise mutation involved is known for that family.

Quantitative assay

The reader is advised to read the introductory chapters of Beutler's practical manual (Beutler, 1984) which contain very useful details concerning the preparation, stability and storage of reagents and calibration of spectrophotometers as well as details of the assay technique. A description of the method recommended by the ICSH (1977) is given in the Appendix.

In the quantitative methods a recording spectrophotometer is helpful but the assay can be undertaken with any spectrophotometer which can measure absorbance at 340 nm and in which the temperature of the cuvette can be maintained within 1–2°C at 30 or 37°C. Since the activity of G6PD is calculated from the change in absorption at 340 nm due to the reduction of NADP to NADPH it is important to know the millimolar extinction coefficient of NADPH in the spectrophotometer being used for the assay. In practice the millimolar extinction coefficient of 6.22 can be used (the absorption of a millimolar solution in a 1 cm cuvette at 340 nm) if the bandwidth of the spectrophotometer is 4 nm or less. If the bandwidth is larger than this it may be necessary to calibrate the spectrophotometer using an accurately prepared solution of NADPH since the extinction coefficient will fall as the bandwidth gets larger. In any case a normal range for a given laboratory (and spectrophotometer) should be established and used for comparison.

Like all enzyme reactions the chemical reactions associated with G6PD are affected by temperature: a higher temperature will lead to an increase in the reaction rate and will therefore appear to give both an increase in activity and an apparent loss of precision if assessed by the standard deviation, but no change in precision if assessed by the coefficient of variation. For the same reason the apparent sensitivity of the tests will increase with temperature. Since the effect of temperature can be significant it is essential that the reaction is undertaken at a known constant temperature and that a 'normal range' is used which has been established at that temperature. Formulae have been drawn up to indicate the effect of temperature on reaction rate (Beutler, 1984) but these should not be relied on in a clinical situation. In practice it is much easier to control the temperature of the cuvette if the temperature chosen is significantly above ambient temperature because most temperature controllers only have heaters and rely on the ambient temperature for cooling.

It is important to remember that the normal range for G6PD activity by the WHO stage method is different from (and higher than) that obtained using the Glock and McLean method (see Appendix).

Characterization of G6PD variants

Although at the present time knowledge of the electrophoretic and functional properties of a G6PD variant rarely affect the clinical management of a patient such studies can be undertaken by special laboratories.

Conclusion

G6PD deficiency is the most common red cell enzymopathy and deficiency of this enzyme has considerable clinical implications. It should be possible for one of the screening tests and the quantitative assays described above to be undertaken by any district laboratory. The reagents are stable and no specialized equipment is required. However, it is necessary to appreciate the limitations of the tests carried out and the circumstances which can lead to difficulties in the interpretation of the results.

Appendix

Fluorescent screening test

International Committee for Standards in Haematology (ICSH, 1979)

REAGENTS

β-NADP	7.5 mmol/l	2 ml	
Glucose-6-phosphate	10 mmol/l	4 ml	
Saponin	10 g/l	4 ml	
Tris-HCl buffer	0.75 mol/l, pH 7.8	6 ml.	It is essential to use a pH electrode which is suitable for Tris.
Oxidized glutathione (GSSG)	8 mmol/l	2 ml	
Distilled water		2 ml	
		20 ml	

Mix the reagents in the volumes stated to make a total volume of 20 ml and then dispense this reaction mixture in 0.2 ml aliquots (in 0.5–1 ml tube) and store frozen at −20°C. This mixture is stable for up to 1 year at this temperature.

BLOOD SAMPLES

Blood may be anticoagulated with EDTA (any sodium or potassium salt) heparin or ACD and dried blood spots collected onto filter paper can also be used. Samples give reliable results even after storage for up to 5 days at 25°C or for up to 21 days at 4°C.

Method

Thaw an aliquot of the reaction mixture and allow it to come to room temperature. Mix 20 μl of whole anticoagulated blood with 0.2 ml of reaction mixture. Spot one drop of this mixture onto non-fluorescent filter paper such as Whatman No. 1, as soon as it has been mixed, and again at intervals of 5 and 10 minutes from the mixing time. Examine the spots under long wavelength UV light as soon as they have dried. (Preferably over a hot plate.)

Note. The presence of GSSG in the reaction mixture increases the sensitivity of the method. This is because the GSSG allows the small amounts of NADPH which may be formed by residual G6PD in mildly deficient samples to be reoxidized by glutathione reductase, another enzyme present in the red cell haemolysate.

Interpretation

At the beginning of the incubation no fluorescence should be visible and the samples from people with normal G6PD activity will fluoresce after 10 minutes incubation. G6PD deficiency is indicated by delayed or absent fluorescence.

Dye decolorization test

Motulsky *et al.* (1959)

REAGENTS

Stored reagents are stable for up to 1 year at the temperatures given.

β-NADP	0.7 mmol/l. Freeze 1 ml aliquots at −20°C
Glucose-6-phosphate	30 mmol/l. Freeze 1 ml aliquots at −20°C
Liquid paraffin	Store at room temperature
Buffer-dye mixture	0.7 mol/l Tris-HCl, pH 8.5, containing 320 mg/l brilliant cresyl blue. Freeze 4.5 ml aliquots at −20°C. It is essential to use a pH electrode which is suitable for Tris
Working mixture	Thaw one aliquot of NADP, G6P and the buffer-dye mixture and mix.

BLOOD SAMPLE

Blood should be anticoagulated with EDTA and used within 24 hours of collection. Make a haemolysate by adding 20 μl of whole blood to 1 ml of water, mix well and use within 6 hours. Always include a control sample with normal G6PD activity and if possible a control sample with reduced G6PD activity.

Method

Add 0.65 ml of the working mixture to the haemolysate, mix and cover with a layer of liquid paraffin. Place in a waterbath at 37°C and record the time for decolorization to occur.

Interpretation

Normal range	35–60 minutes
G6PD deficiency	1.5–24 hours

Note. In very anaemic subjects (PCV less than 0.25) adjust the PCV to 0.4–0.5 before making the haemolysate.

Cytochemical assay

Fairbanks and Lampe (1968)

REAGENTS:

Sodium chloride	0.15 mol/l
Sodium chloride	0.1 mol/l
Sodium nitrite	0.18 mol/l
MTT*	5 mg/ml
Incubation mixture	Mix the following reagents so that the mixture will have the final concentration stated and divide into 1 ml aliquots which are stable for 3 weeks at 4°C or for at least 1 year at −20°C Glucose (28 mmol/l), Phosphate buffer (50 mmol, pH 7.0) Sodium chloride (58 mmol/l), and Nile blue sulphate (11 mg/l)

BLOOD SAMPLES

It is best to use blood anticoagulated in ACD (5 ml of blood in 1 ml of ACD) which can be used for up to 1 week after collection. Heparinized and EDTA blood samples can also be used, but must be used on the day of venesection to avoid excessive crenation.

Procedure

1 Centrifuge sample, remove the supernatant plasma and add 0.5 ml of packed red cells to a centrifuge tube containing 9 ml 0.15 mol/l sodium chloride and 0.5 ml of 0.18 mol/l sodium nitrite. Incubate undisturbed at 37°C for 20 minutes.
2 Centrifuge at 4°C for 15 minutes at 550 g. Remove and discard the supernatant without disturbing the buffy coat.
3 Wash the red cells three times with 9 ml of cold 0.15 mol/l sodium chloride at 4°C as in step 2 above. After each wash remove the buffy coat taking care to remove as few red cells as possible.
4 Mix the packed RBC and transfer 50 μl to a tube containing 1 ml of the incubation mixture.
Incubate undisturbed at 37°C for 30 minutes.
5 Add 0.2 ml of MTT and resuspend the red cells by gentle agitation. Continue the incubation at 37°C for a further 60 minutes.
6 Resuspend the red cells thoroughly and mix one drop of this suspension with one drop of 0.1 mol/l sodium chloride on a microscope slide and cover with a coverslip.
7 Within 30 minutes of making the preparation examine 500 red cells with a ×100 oil immersion objective and score their granularity as follows:

No granules	0
1–3 granules	1+
4–6 granules	2+
More than 7 granules	3+

Interpretation

In subjects with normal G6PD activity most of the red cells will contain some granules and more than 30% will score 3+. In deficient hemizygous males less than 20% of the red cells

*MTT = 3–(4,5–dimethylthiazolyl–2)–2, 5 diphenyltetrazolium bromide.

will contain any granules. Mosaicism in heterozygous females should be easy to recognize since one population will have normal granules and the other population will have few or no granules. The results are often easier to interpret if they are plotted as a bar graph.

G6PD quantitative assay

See Beutler (1984)

REAGENTS

These may be stored at the temperatures given for up to 1 year.

β-NADP	2 mmol/l. Freeze 2 ml aliquots at −20°C
Glucose-6-phosphate	6 mmol/l. Freeze 1 ml aliquots at −20°C
6-phosphogluconate	6 mmol/l. Freeze 1 ml aliquots at −20°C
Magnesium chloride	0.1 mol/l. Store at 4°C
Sodium chloride	0.15 mol/l. Store at 4°C
Tris-HCl, 1 mol/l, EDTA 5 mmol/l, pH 8.0	Store at 4°C It is essential to use a pH electrode which is suitable for Tris
Haemolysing reagent	Mix 0.05 ml of β-mercaptoethanol and 10 ml of neutralized 10% (0.27 mol/l) EDTA and make up to 1 litre with water

BLOOD SAMPLES

Blood samples may be anticoagulated with EDTA, heparin or ACD and give reliable results after storage at 5 days at 25°C or 21 days at 4°C.

Haemolysate

Filtration of whole, anticoagulated blood through a mixed cellulose column to remove white cells and platelets is preferable (Beutler, 1984), but if this is not practical centrifugation of the blood and removal of the plasma and buffy coat is satisfactory.

Wash the red cells twice in cold 0.15 mol/l sodium chloride and then resuspend the red cells in an equal volume of cold 0.15 mol/l sodium chloride. Add 0.2 ml of the cell suspension to 1.8 ml of the haemolysing reagent. Freeze and thaw the haemolysate by placing the tube containing the haemolysate in an ice-alcohol mixture until it is frozen and then thaw by placing the tube in a beaker of water at room temperature. Next measure the haemoglobin concentration. This haemolysate should be kept cold (preferably in ice) and should be used within 2 hours. Removal of the stroma is not necessary.

Procedure

The reagents shown in Table A1 are added to cuvettes with a critical volume of less than 1 ml. If cuvettes with a critical volume of less than 3 ml are used the volumes of all the reagents must be multiplied by three.

Mix, incubate at constant temperature (30° or 37°C) and record the absorbance of

Table A1

	Cuvette			
	1	2	3	4
Tris-HC1, EDTA buffer	100*	100	100	100
$MgC1_2$	100	100	100	100
NADP	100	100	100	100
Water	680	580	580	480
Haemolysate	20	20	20	20
Mix and incubate at constant temperature for 10 minutes				
G-6-P	—	100	—	100
6-PGA	—	—	100	100

* μl.

the cuvettes at 340 nm for 15 minutes. The recorder should have a full scale expansion of 1.0 A.

The reaction rate and, therefore, the rate of increase in absorbance at 340 nm, usually increases for the first few minutes, then becomes linear and finally slows down as the substrates are used up.

Use the linear part of the curve for the calculation. Draw a straight line through the recorded points then read off the increase in absorbance over a 10 minute period and divide by 10 to obtain the increase in one minute (ΔA).

Calculation

Enzyme activity in iu/gHb

$$= \frac{\text{change in absorbance at 340 nm/minute}}{6.22} \times \text{dilution factor} \times \frac{100}{\text{Hb}}$$

Where the 'Hb' = Hb concentration of the haemolysate in g/dl. In the method given above this can be simplified to:

G6PD (WHO method)

$$= \frac{\Delta A(\text{cuvette 2–cuvette 1}) \times 804}{\text{Hb concentration of haemolysate (g/dl)}} \text{iu/gHb}$$

G6PD (Glock & McLean method)

$$= \frac{\Delta A(\text{cuvette 4–cuvette 3}) \times 804}{\text{Hb concentration of haemolysate (g/dl)}} \text{iu/gHb}$$

$$6PGD = \frac{\Delta A(\text{cuvette 3–cuvette 1}) \times 804}{\text{Hb concentration of haemolysate (g/dl)}} \text{iu/gHb}$$

Where ΔA = change in absorbance in 1 minute.

Normal values (mean ± 2SD at 37°C)

G6PD (WHO method) 12.1 ± 4.2 iu/gHb

G6PD (Glock & McLean method)	8.3 ± 3.2
6PGD	8.8 ± 1.7

It is important for each laboratory to establish its own normal ranges and to include a normal control sample with each assay.

Interpretation

The Glock and McLean method (cuvettes 4–3) is usually a more accurate expression of the true G6PD activity than the WHO method (cuvette 2–1). However, at very low enzyme activities this involves subtracting a large, experimentally determined value (G6PD, cuvette 3), from a slightly larger one (G6PD + 6PGD, cuvette 4). In this situation the WHO method (cuvette 2–1) is preferred.

References

Beutler E. (1971) Abnormalities of the hexose monophosphate shunt. *Seminars in Haematology* **VIII**, 311–347.

Beutler E. (1984) *Red Cell Metabolism, A Manual of Biochemical Methods* 3rd edn, Grune and Stratton, Orlando.

Dacie J.V. (1985) *The Haemolytic Anaemias* 3rd edn, Part I, pp. 365–419. Churchill Livingstone, Edinburgh.

Fairbanks V.F. & Lampe L.T. (1968) ‘A tetrazolium-linked cytochemical method for estimation of glucose-6-phosphate dehydrogenase activity in individual erythrocytes: applications in the study of heterozygotes for glucose-6-phosphate dehydrogenase deficiency’. *Blood* **31**, 589.

Glock G.E. & McLean P. (1953) Further studies on properties and assay of glucose-6-phosphate dehydrogenase and 6-phosphogluconate dehydrogenase of rat liver. *Biochemical Journal* **55**, 400–408.

Grimes A.J. (1980) *Human Red Cell Metabolism* pp. 239–258. Blackwell Scientific Publications, Oxford.

Herz F., Kaplan E. & Scheye E.S. (1970) Diagnosis of erythrocyte glucose-6-phosphate dehydrogenase deficiency in the Negro male despite haemolytin crisis. *Blood* **35**, 90.

ICSH (1977) Recommended methods for red-cell enzyme analysis. *British Journal of Haematology* **35**, 331.

ICSH (1979) Recommended screening test for glucose-6-phosphate dehydrogenase (G-6-PD) deficiency. *British Journal of Haematology* **43**, 469.

Lewis S.M. & Saunders K.J. (1989) Screening for G6PD by sigma kits. *Clinical and Laboratory Haematology* **11**, 76–78.

Luzzatto L. & Mehta A.B. (1989) *The Metabolic Basis of Inherited Disease* 6th edn, p. 2245. McGraw-Hill, New York.

Motulsky A.G., Kraut J.M. Thieme W.T. & Musto D.F. (1959) Biochemical genetics of glucose-6-phosphate deficiency. *Clinical Research* **7**, 89–90.

Scriver C., Beaudet A., Sly W. & Valle D. (1989) *The Metabolic Basis of Inherited Disease.* 6th edn, p. 2245. McGraw-Hill, New York.

Report of a WHO Scientific Group (1967) Standardization of procedures for the study of glucose-6-phosphate dehydrogenase. *World Health Organization Technical Report Series* **366**.

Wintrobe M.M. (1981) *Clinical Haematology*, 8th edn, pp. 786–795. Lea and Febiger, Philadelphia.

8 Oral Anticoagulation

Prepared by the
Haemostasis and Thrombosis Task Force

Introduction

The guidelines document on oral anticoagulation first appeared in 1984. Since then the international system for the standardization of the prothrombin time in anticoagulant control, based on International Normalized Ratios (INR), has become widely accepted (Lewis, 1987; Shinton, 1983; Loeliger *et al.*, 1985). The introduction of INR, combined with the change in the UK from human brain to rabbit thromboplastin in 1986, has created a need for this update.

A survey on oral anticoagulation conducted for the British Society for Haematology (BSH) via the United Kingdom National External Quality Assessment Scheme (NEQAS) in blood coagulation in 1982 estimated that 2.3 million prothrombin time tests were performed annually in the UK for purposes of oral anticoagulant control and that about a quarter of a million people were receiving this treatment each year. The numbers are now much greater.

Properties of oral anticoagulants

The commonly used oral anticoagulant drugs are those derived from 4-hydroxycoumarin, of which the most widely used is warfarin, named after the Wisconsin Alumni Research Foundation. Other drugs listed in the *British National Formulary* are nicoumalone and phenindione. Phenindione is now rarely used due to hypersensitivity reactions.

Oral anticoagulants antagonize vitamin K, required for the gamma carboxylation of certain glutamic acid residues which facilitate calcium binding of coagulation factors II, VII, IX, X and the anticoagulant factors protein C and protein S. Acarboxy forms which circulate in patients treated with coumarin drugs are devoid of procoagulant properties. The rate of disappearance from the circulation of these vitamin K dependent clotting factors depends on their respective half lives, which range from six to 60 hours.

Reprinted with permission from the *Journal of Clinical Pathology*, 1990 **43**, 177–183.

Use of oral anticoagulants

Coumarin drugs are used for the prevention and control of thrombo-embolism. The following are the conditions for which oral anticoagulants are used, but there are wide differences of opinion on their indications.

Short term to medium term (up to 12 months)

Prophylaxis of deep vein thrombosis including high risk surgery (Sevitt, 1962; Taberner *et al.*, 1978; Francis *et al.*, 1983); myocardial infarction, anterior myocardial infarction, 3 months minimum (Resenekow *et al.*, 1989); established deep vein thrombosis, 3 months minimum (Hyers *et al.*, 1989); xenograft heart valve replacements, 3 months minimum (Stein & Kantrowitz, 1989); pulmonary embolism, 3–6 months (Hyers *et al.*, 1989); coronary artery bypass graft, up to 2 months (Gohlke *et al.*, 1981).

Long term

Recurrent venous thrombo-embolism (Hyers *et al.*, 1989); embolic complications of rheumatic heart disease and atrial fibrillation (Petersen *et al.*, 1989); cardiac prosthetic valve replacement and arterial grafts (Stein & Kantrowitz, 1989; Hirsh *et al.*, 1989).

POSSIBLE INDICATIONS FOR LONG TERM TREATMENT

Congenital antithrombin III deficiency with clinical thrombosis; congenital protein C or S deficiencies with clinical thrombosis; transient ischaemic cerebral artery syndrome including basilar and vertebral artery syndromes; lupus-like anticoagulant with clinical thrombosis.

Pregnancy

The decision on whether to use oral anticoagulant drugs during pregnancy is still a matter of clinical judgement because of the balance of risk between mother and fetus.

The main disadvantage of vitamin K antagonists during pregnancy is that they cross the placenta. Warfarin may be teratogenic during the first trimester, resulting in warfarin embryopathy, and is associated with an increasing risk of fetal haemorrhage as pregnancy progresses. The risk is maximal during labour and delivery. A warning on the dangers of becoming pregnant while taking oral anticoagulants is given in the national anticoagulant treatment booklet.

When anticoagulation during pregnancy is deemed essential, intravenous or self-administered subcutaneous heparin in adjusted doses should be considered. (For further details of heparin administration see BSH guidelines on heparin). Long term heparin administration, however, carries a risk of maternal osteoporosis. Women who have prosthetic heart valves or who have mitral valve disease or atrial fibrillation, or both, may be more safely maintained on warfarin. Wherever possible, oral anticoagulants should be avoided during the first trimester. In any patient given warfarin during the second and third trimesters frequent monitoring and dose review are essential. For all patients warfarin must be replaced by heparin at around 36 weeks.

If heparin is continued during labour its dose should be carefully monitored. After delivery full dose heparin may usually be reintroduced 12–24 hours after completion of the third stage. Oral anticoagulants may be given 24–48 hours after delivery. Introduction of vitamin K antagonists should be progressive, with no initial loading dose. Heparin should be continued until the INR is in the desired therapeutic range. Anticoagulated mothers of healthy infants should not be discouraged from breast feeding.

Contraindications

These are seldom absolute and depend on individual patients (see below).

General	Mental impairment Uncooperative patients Alcoholism
Cardiovascular	Hypertension
Renal	Sustained increase of blood urea above 10 μmol/litre
Neurological	Recent non-embolic cerebrovascular accidents, recent surgery, or trauma to central nervous system and eye
Gastrointestinal	Inflammatory bowel disease, peptic ulcer, oesophageal varices
Liver disease	Uncompensated cirrhosis
Haematological	Pre-existing haemostatic defect

Dose and control of anticoagulant treatment

The dose of anticoagulant drug depends on biological assay of the induced coagulation defect, measured by the prothrombin time, which is the recalcification time of plasma after the addition of a tissue thromboplastin. Thromboplastin reagents derive from a variety of sources and usually give different prothrombin times for the same test plasma because of differing potencies and responsiveness to depression of the vitamin K dependent clotting factors. All thromboplastin reagents should be labelled with an International Sensitivity Index (ISI) which quantifies their responsiveness to the effects of anticoagulants in terms of the WHO Primary Reference Preparation which has an assigned value of 1.0. This permits reporting as INR. INR are virtually identical with the formerly recommended British Ratios (BR) (Loeliger *et al.*, 1985).

After clinical appraisal a baseline prothrombin time should be determined whenever possible to assess liver function before the initial dose of warfarin is administered. The usual adult induction dose of warfarin is 10 mg on the first day and 10 mg on the second day (a larger loading dose is not now recommended).

The dose schedule should be reduced in the following conditions: prolonged baseline prothrombin time; abnormal liver function tests; congestive cardiac failure; parenteral feeding; less than average body weight; age of over 80 years.

The daily dose should be given, if possible, at a fixed time—for example, 1800 hours. The INR must be determined on the day of treatment and the dose of warfarin adjusted accordingly. The maintenance dose is usually between 3 and 9 mg warfarin, although the pharmacological response varies widely among patients and even in the same patient over a period of treatment. If the patient is receiving concurrent heparin treatment by continuous infusion and is being maintained by the activated partial thromboplastin time (APTT) at less than two and a half times control reading (see BSH guidelines on heparin treatment), oral anticoagulant dose can still be based on the prothrombin time from a specimen collected without discontinuing heparin infusion. The prothrombin time prolongation by heparin at therapeutic concentrations is slight. If the dose of heparin is excessive it may be necessary to withhold treatment for 3 to 4 hours and repeat the test. Repeat prothrombin times are normally required daily or on alternate days in the early days of treatment, or at longer intervals later, depending on the response. If a patient is well stabilized the interval of prothrombin time testing can be gradually extended to 8 weeks as an outpatient. Where there is a pronounced change in the clinical state or in concomitant drug treatment, especially if the drug is known to interact with warfarin, the prothrombin time must be checked more frequently. When a known potentiating or antagonizing drug is administered or withdrawn, the dose of warfarin should either be adjusted or the prothrombin time checked more frequently. Other drugs which are recognized as possibly synergistic with oral anticoagulants can be given in normal doses but with more frequent monitoring.

Therapeutic ranges

As experience of the improved anticoagulant control in the UK afforded by the provision of standardized low ISI (high sensitivity) thromboplastin and external quality assessment has increased, more specific and, in some instances, more intense therapeutic ranges have been used with confidence. The BSH proposals (Table 8.1) were based on the results of a NEQAS survey on current practice, supported in respect of prevention and treatment of deep vein thrombosis by previous randomized clinical trials (Sevitt, 1962; Taberner *et al.*, 1978; Francis *et al.*, 1983).

Although surgical procedures, including dental extractions, may be associated with an increased risk of bleeding if these are performed under anticoagulant cover, two randomized studies (Taberner *et al.*, 1978; Francis *et al.*, 1983) have shown that the bleeding risk is low if the INR on the day of operation is between 2.0 and 2.5 with a low ISI thromboplastin. In practice an INR of not greater than 2.0 is recommended at the time of surgery but the risk of bleeding depends on the clinical circumstances.

Side effects

Apart from haemorrhage, side effects encountered with oral anticoagulants have been mostly with the indanediones, principally phenindione, the use of which has been largely discontinued as sensitivity reactions were relatively common. Skin rashes and alopecia have been reported as rare complications with coumarin drugs. Cutaneous necrosis associated in some cases with heterozygous protein C or protein S deficiency is due to capillary thrombosis during the induction phase. In such patients administration of heparin during the first few days of treatment

Table 8.1 Suggested INR ranges in various conditions

INR	Clinical state
2.0–2.5	Prophylaxis of deep vein thrombosis including surgery on high risk patients (Sevitt, 1962; Frances *et al.*, 1983) (2.0–3.0 for hip surgery and fractured femur operations) (Hirsh *et al.*, 1989)
2.0–3.0	Treatment of deep vein thrombosis (Hull *et al.*, 1982) Pulmonary embolism Systemic embolism (Hirsh *et al.*, 1989) Prevention of venous thrombo-embolism in myocardial infarction (Medical Research Council, 1969; Veterans Administration, 1973) Mitral stenosis with embolism (Hirsh *et al.*, 1989) Transient ischaemic attacks Atrial fibrillation (Hirsh *et al.*, 1989)
3.0–4.5	Recurrent deep vein thrombosis and pulmonary embolism (Hirsh *et al.*, 1989) Arterial disease including myocardial infarction (Sixty-Plus Reinfarction Study Group, 1980) Mechanical prosthetic heart valves* (Hirsh *et al.*, 1989)

* A recent randomized study in patients with tissue prosthetic heart valves indicated that control at a less intensive INR range of 2.0–3.0 was effective and safe. (Turpie *et al.*, 1988)

with slow induction of warfarin is advised. Poor control may give similar problems at a later stage in these patients. Demineralization of bone has been reported with prolonged oral anticoagulant treatment in young children. Acute intestinal obstruction is a rare complication of mesenteric haemorrhage.

Causes of prolonged prothrombin time and haemorrhage

These are due to relative overdose or increased sensitivity by the patient either as a consequence of a change in patient's physical state–any severe illness, interaction with a potentiating drug, and withdrawal of antagonistic drugs.

The following pathological disorders have a confirmed potentiating effect: alcohol excess, either acute or chronic; cardiac failure; cholestasis; diarrhoea (enteritis); fever; gastrocolic fistula; hypoalbuminaemia; liver damage (including exposure to organic solvents such as petrol and possibly halothane in general anaesthesia); malnutrition; severe weight reduction regimens; renal impairment; thyrotoxicosis.

Drugs used for the following have a high potentiating effect:

Gastrointestinal tract: Cimetidine.

Cardiovascular system: Amiodarone, clofibrate, bezafibrate, dextrothyroxine, quinidine, sulphinpyrazone.

Infections: Co-trimoxazole, metronidazole.

Endocrine system: Anabolic steroids, danazol, glucagon, thyroxine.

Musculoskeletal and joint disease: Aspirin and the salicylates, azapropazone, feprazone, sulphinpyrazone.

Malignant disease: Tamoxifen.

Alcoholism: Disulfiram.

A fuller list of drugs available in the UK which may potentiate or antagonize anticoagulants is given in the Appendix.

Recommendations for concomitant drug treatment

Analgesics used for headaches and minor trauma containing dextropropoxyphene hydrochloride or paracetamol, or a combination with co-proxamol, (Distalgesic), are relatively safe for occasional self-medication in doses of two to four tablets a day, once or twice a week, but regular ingestion of six to eight tablets daily for chronic pain may require reduction of oral anticoagulant dose.

While most interacting drugs operate by potentiating or antagonizing the action of coumarin-like drugs, others, such as aspirin, sulphinpyrazone, and non-steroidal anti-inflammatory drugs, also act by impairing platelet function and so enhance the risk of bleeding, especially in the gastrointestinal tract. Aspirin also has an undesirable localized irritant effect on the gastric mucosa, resulting in an increased incidence of haematemesis. Thus prothrombin time control alone will not reflect the potential risk of bleeding.

Reversal of oral anticoagulant treatment

Recommendations on reversal of oral anticoagulant treatment have to be influenced by the risks of inducing hepatitis and human immunodeficiency virus (HIV) infection with plasma concentrates and the possible thrombotic dangers of over correction by vitamin K, especially in patients with prosthetic or replacement heart valves (Table 8.2). With these risks in mind, the following recommendations are made with the warning that 4 to 6 hours must be allowed for an adequate clinical response to vitamin K_1 in the average patient.

Table 8.2 Recommendations on reversal of oral anticoagulant treatment

Life threatening haemorrhage
Immediately give 5 mg vitamin K_1 by slow intravenous infusion and a concentrate of factor II, IX, X, with factor VII concentrate (if available)
The dose of concentrate should be calculated based on 50 iu factor IX/kg body weight
If no concentrate is available fresh frozen plasma should be infused (about 1 litre for an adult) but this may not be as effective

Less severe haemorrhage such as haematuria and epistaxis
Withhold warfarin for one or more days and consider giving vitamin K_1 0.5–2.0 mg intravenously

INR of > 4.5 without haemorrhage
Withdraw warfarin for one or two days then review

Unexpected bleeding at therapeutic levels
Investigate possibility of underlying cause such as unsuspected renal or alimentary tract disease

Causes of INR of less than 2.0

Failure to achieve an adequate degree of anticoagulation may be due to inadequate dose, patient non-compliance, hereditary resistance, acquired resistance to warfarin, improvement in the patient's general condition, dietary changes or antagonistic drug interaction. Plasma warfarin concentration may assist in diagnosis of non-compliance. Barbiturates and preparations containing vitamin K are particularly prone to cause low INR values; other drugs prescribed in the UK that are antagonistic to oral anticoagulants are listed in the Appendix. Acquired drug resistance, although a rare occurrence, may be difficult to manage. Changing to an alternative drug may be beneficial, but resistance is often encountered with other oral anticoagulant compounds.

Withdrawal of oral anticoagulant treatment

Whether treatment should be withdrawn abruptly or gradually withdrawn ('tailed off') is still debatable. Theoretically, the 'rebound hypercoagulability' which results from sudden discontinuation might predispose to rebound thrombosis. Some clinicians tail off long term treatment over several weeks but withdraw short term treatment suddenly.

Organization of oral anticoagulant control service

Each haematology service or department should provide a clinical and laboratory service for the control of oral anticoagulant treatment. This should be concerned solely with the supervision of anticoagulant doses and related problems. Prescription of oral anticoagulant drugs must be the responsibility of a registered medical practitioner.

INPATIENT SERVICE

The consultant haematologist should be willing to advise on the hospital's policy for the control of oral anticoagulant drugs. He or she should provide advice on the selection of patients and the appropriate therapeutic range and should counsel patients on oral anticoagulant drugs. A survey on oral anticoagulation conducted for the British Society for Haematology through the United Kingdom National External Quality Assessment Scheme (NEQAS) indicated that half of inpatient anticoagulant control is undertaken by consultant haematologists alone or with junior haematology staff. In some additional instances responsibility is shared with consultant colleagues. Where anticoagulant treatment gets out of control or requires to be reversed, the haematologist should advise on measures to correct this and provide blood products as necessary.

The haematologist should organize a laboratory service for the control of oral anticoagulant drugs according to the principles set out in these guidelines. There should be formal referral in writing of patients to the anticoagulant clinic with treatment authorization signed by the requesting medical practitioner. For inpatient doses, this will normally be based on the prothrombin time of venous blood samples sent to the laboratory. Written reports giving INR values should be issued and the results entered in the ward, into an anticoagulant control chart.

OUTPATIENT SERVICE

Patients on discharge from hospital should normally be referred to a consultant haematologist for the control of outpatient treatment. Each haematology department or service should be prepared to organize outpatient clinics for the control of oral anticoagulant drugs and where possible should provide laboratory services at these clinics to enable dose adjustment to be made on the spot (advising on dose by telephone is to be avoided). The work of these clinics should be confined to the supervision and regulation of anticoagulant dose and related problems. A capillary blood prothrombin time technique is useful for outpatient clinics as it reduces the overall time for testing.

A request to the haematologist for anticoagulant supervision and dose should be in writing and should be signed. An outpatient anticoagulant request card giving patient details and proposed duration of treatment, together with the list of drugs given concomitantly, ideally should be provided with each request.

Patients should be issued with national anticoagulant booklets for the recording of INR results and anticoagulant dose. Supplies of these booklets are available from: DHSS Stores, No. 2 Site, Manchester Road, Heywood, Lancashire, OL10 2PZ, or SHHD (Div. IIID), Room 9, St Andrews House, Edinburgh, EH1 3DE. There should be regular correspondence between the clinic doctor and the patient's general practitioner. The practitioner should be informed of non-attendance, any problems associated with treatment, and of a decision to withdraw treatment.

Outpatient anticoagulant clinics should be staffed by adequate numbers of medical, nursing, scientific and secretarial staff. Full records of patients' attendances, results, anticoagulant dosing and correspondence should be kept in special anticoagulant clinic case records.

The dose should also be recorded in the patient's booklet and on the local record. This information should ideally be conveyed to the patient while in the anticoagulant clinic but where for logistic reasons this is not possible, the recorded dose in the booklet should be posted to the patient as soon as possible.

QUALITY CONTROL OF ANTICOAGULANT ADMINISTRATION

This should be carried out either by determining the proportion of patients within their relevant therapeutic range or by determining the mean percentage adequately treated, with the coefficient of variation (CV) for each therapeutic range. More detailed therapeutic quality control has been advocated in which assessment of the effective ratio for control defined as the mid-point between two estimations is determined (Duxbury, 1982).

Laboratory control of oral anticoagulants

STANDARDIZATION OF THE PROTHROMBIN TIME IN ANTICOAGULANT CONTROL

The coagulation defect induced by oral anticoagulant treatment is best quantified by the INR. The INR is the prothrombin ratio which, it is calculated, would have been obtained with the WHO primary international reference preparation.

INTERNATIONAL REFERENCE PREPARATIONS (IRP)

The primary WHO international reference thromboplastin—human brain 67/40 combined—was replaced by a second WHO IRP of human brain plain, British Comparative Thromboplastin batch 253 (1983). Additional IRP of rabbit brain plain (RBT/79) and bovine combined (OBT/79) were approved by the WHO in the same year.

CALIBRATION OF THROMBOPLASTIN REAGENTS

An orthogonal regression analysis is the recommended WHO procedure to compare different thromboplastin reagents and derive equivalent INR. A rectilinear relation of the logarithms of the prothrombin times is used. The slope of the correlation indicates the correlation of the local thromboplastin with the IRP (Lewis, 1987; Shinton, 1983; Loeliger *et al.*, 1985; Kirkwood, 1983; Tomensen & Thomson, 1985). This is termed the International Sensitivity Index (ISI). IRP results are plotted on the vertical axis against the logarithms of prothrombin times obtained with the thromboplastin to be calibrated on the same set of plasmas (from 20 normal subjects and 60 stable anticoagulated patients). An ISI can be assigned to each batch of thromboplastin. Prothrombin time results should be given as INR, which may be derived from one of the following formulae, when the ISI is known.

$$\text{INR} = \text{antilog}\ (\log\ (\text{prothrombin ratio}) \times \text{ISI})$$

or

$$\text{INR} = (\text{prothrombin ratio})^{\text{ISI}}$$

With some reagents, INR values are reliably obtained from a chart produced by the manufacturer, but with others they are derived from one of the above equations. To determine the normal control value the NEQAS Steering Committee in Blood Coagulation has recommended that the geometric mean of a minimum of 20 normal controls should be used. The normal control values should be obtained from healthy ambulant adults, men and women, and need not necessarily be tested on one day. A locally determined geometric normal mean should be compared with the mean normal value for each batch of thromboplastin issued by the manufacturer, and this may be used to determine the INR. In view of the heavy demands and complexity of the procedure, ISI calibrations should not normally be performed by routine hospital laboratories and should only be performed by National Control Laboratories or by manufacturers. The ISI calibration procedure is described in detail elsewhere (Kirkwood, 1983; Tomensen & Thomson, 1985).

THE CLINICAL IMPORTANCE OF A LOW ISI THROMBOPLASTIN

The recommended BSH therapeutic ranges have been based on clinical trials and cumulative experience in the UK with thromboplastins of ISI between 1.0 and 1.1. NEQAS surveys have shown that these give a lower incidence of persistent poor performance and a lower CV of the INR—that is, increased precision (Poller *et al.*, 1988). Of clinical importance is that the width of the therapeutic range diminishes progressively with increasing ISI (see Fig. 8.1).

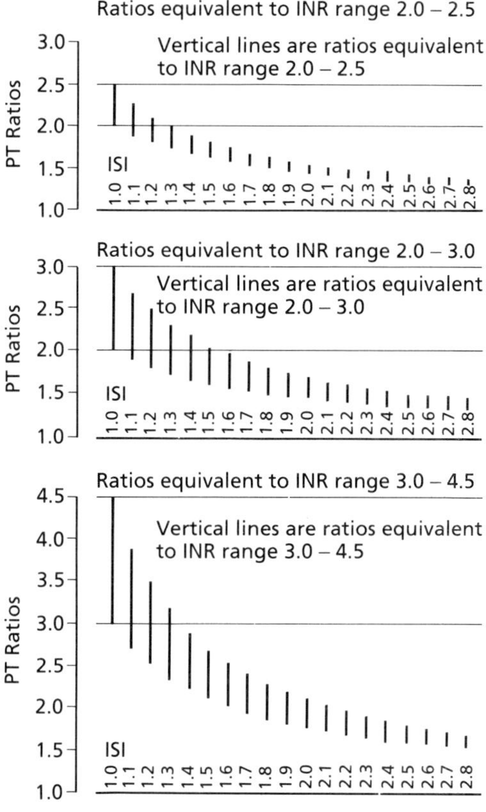

Fig. 8.1 Therapeutic prothrombin ratios equivalent to INR ranges related to increasing ISI of thromboplastins. PT ratios are given for each ISI.

The INR value may also be less dependable with higher ISI reagents in the induction period of oral anticoagulation and in unstabilized patients.

USE OF COAGULOMETERS

ISI determinations are based on prothrombin time values obtained with a manual technique. According to 1988 NEQAS data, almost 50% of UK prothrombin times are performed using a coagulometer. Coagulometers affect the INR value to varying degrees. NEQAS surveys indicate that most types of coagulometer tend to underestimate the INR whereas a minority overestimate the INR. There is, however, considerable variation in performance with instruments of the same model which means that it is not generally safe to apply an ISI correction factor for a type of coagulometer or coagulometer/reagent system as each instrument must be checked individually.

CONTROL BY CHROMOGENIC (AMIDOLYTIC) SUBSTRATES

Amidolytic assays based on synthetic chromogenic substrates have been recommended for oral anticoagulant dose control. The chromogenic assays are relatively specific to one clotting factor and may measure acarboxy forms. No single chromogenic substrate technique seems to be satisfactory for the control of short-term anticoagulant administration, but specific factor II, VII, and factor X chromogenic methods give a reasonable approximation to the prothrombin time in long-term stabilized patients (O'Donnell *et al.*, 1983).

USE OF COMPUTERS

Computers may play a valuable part in patient records, administration of clinic appointments, and analysis of therapeutic quality control. Their value in production of dose schedules for individual patients is under investigation. Their use for the latter cannot yet be recommended until reliable patient databased programmes have been developed.

Appendix

Drugs reported as interacting with oral anticoagulants

The preparations listed in Table A1 should not be regarded as contraindicated or as contraindications to warfarin administration. Their prescription may, however, cause changes in oral anticoagulant requirements. Caution is therefore advised and more frequent monitoring may be required. This list is not intended to be comprehensive. Some drugs have only been referred to in single case reports.

Table A1

	Potentiating drugs	Antagonistic drugs
Gastrointestinal tract	Antacids—magnesium salts Cimetidine Liquid paraffin and other laxatives	Chloestyramine Colestipol
Cardiovascular system	Amiodarone Clofibrate Dextrothyroxine Diazoxide Dipyridamole Ethacrynic acid Quinindine Sulphinpyrazone	Cholestyramine Colestipol Spironolactone
Respiratory system		Antihistamines
Central nervous system	Chloral hydrate and related compounds Chlorpromazine Dextropropoxyphene Dichloralphenazone—initial Diflunisal Mefenamic acid Monoamine oxidase inhibitors Tricyclic antidepressants Triclofos sodium	Barbiturates Carbamazepine Dichloralphenazone—late Haloperidol Phenytoin Primidone

Infections	Aminoglycosides
	  Amikacin
	  Gentamicin
	  Kanamycin
	  Neomycin
	  Streptomycin
	  Tobramycin
	Co-trimoxazole
	Cephalosporins
	  Cephaloridine
	  Cephazolin
	  Cephamandole
	  Latamoxef
	Chloramphenicol
	Cycloserine
	Erythromycin
	Isoniazid
	Ketoconazole
	Metronidazole
	Miconazole
	Nalidixic acid
	Penicillin G—large doses—intravenous
	Ampicillin—oral
	Quinine salts
		Griseofulvin
		Rifampicin

Table A1 (cont'd)

	Potentiating drugs	Antagonistic drugs
Infections (cont'd)	Streptotriad	
	Sulphonamides—long acting	
	Tetracycline	
Endocrine system	Anabolic steroids	Oral contraceptives
	Chlorpropamide	
	Corticosteroids	
	Danazol	
	Glucagon	
	Metoclopramide	
	Propylthiouracil	
	Sulphonyl urea	
	Thyroxine	
	Tolbutamide	
Malignant disease and immunosuppression	Cyclophosphamide	
	Mercaptopurine	
	Methotrexate	
	Immunosuppressant drugs	
	Tamoxifen	
Musculoskeletal and joint disease	Allopurinol	
	Aspirin and the salicylates	
	Azapropazone	
	Diflunisal	
	Fenclofenac	
	Fenoprofen	
	Feprazone	
	Flufenamic acid	
	Flurbiprofen	
	Indomethacin	
	Ketoprofen	
	Mefenamic acid	
	Naproxen	
	Paracetamol—high daily doses (with dextropropoxyphene Distalgesic/ coproxamol)	
	Piroxicam	
	Sulindac	
	Sulphinpyrazone	
Nutrition and blood	Alcohol—dose dependent potentiator	Vitamin K Alcohol
Ear, nose and oesophagus		Antihistamines Phenazone
Skin		Antihistamines
Alcoholism	Disulfiram (Antabuse)	

References

Duxbury B. McD. (1982) Therapeutic control of anticoagulant treatment. *British Medical Journal* **284**, 702.

Francis C.W., Marder V.J., McCollister E.C. *et al.* (1983) Two step warfarin therapy. *Journal of the American Medical Association* **249**, 374–398.

Gohlke H., Gohlke-Barwolf C., Sturzenhofecker P. *et al.* (1981) Improved graft patency with anticoagulant therapy after coronary artery bypass surgery: a prospective randomized study. *Circulation* **64** (Suppl. II), 22–27.

Hirsh J., Poller L., Deykin D. *et al.* (1989) Optimal therapeutic range for oral anticoagulants. *Chest* **95**, 5S–11S.

Hull R., Hirsh J., Jay R. *et al.* (1982) Different intensities of oral anticoagulant therapy in the treatment of proximal-vein thrombosis. *New England Journal of Medicine* **307**, 1676.

Hyers T.S., Hull R.D. & Weg J.C. (1989) Antithrombotic therapy for venous thromboembolic disease. *Chest* **95**, 37S–51S.

Kirkwood T.B.L. (1983) Calibration of reference thromboplastins and standardisation of the prothrombin ratio. *Thrombosis and Haemostasis* **49**, 238–244.

Lewis S.M. (1987) Thromboplastin and oral anticoagulant control. *British Journal of Haematology* **66**, 1–4.

Loeliger E.A., Poller L., Samama M. *et al.* (1985) Questions and answers on prothrombin time standardisation in oral anticoagulant control. *Thrombosis and Haemostasis* **54**, 515–517.

Medical Research Council (1969) Assessment of short term anticoagulant administration after cardiac infarction. *British Medical Journal* **1**, 1335–1342.

O'Donnell J.R., Walker I.D., Davidson J.F. (1983) Control of oral anticoagulant therapy with a chromogenic prothrombin assay. *British Journal of Haematology* **55**, 172–175.

Petersen P., Boysen G., Godtfredsen J. *et al.* (1989) Placebo controlled randomised trial of warfarin and aspirin for prevention of thromboembolic complications in chronic atrial fibrillation. *Lancet* **i**, 175–178.

Poller L., Taberner D.A., Thomson J.M. & Darby K.V. (1988) Survey of prothrombin time results in National External Quality Assessment Scheme exercises 1980–87. *Journal of Clinical Pathology* **48**, 361–364.

Resenekow L., Chediak J., Hirsh J. & Lewis H.D. (1989) Antithrombotic agents in coronary heart disease. *Chest* **95**, 52S–72S.

Sevitt S. (1962) Venous thrombosis and pulmonary embolism. Their prevention by oral anticoagulation. *American Journal of Medicine* **33**, 703.

Shinton N.K. (1983) Standardisation of oral anticoagulant therapy. *British Medical Journal* **287**, 1000–1001.

Sixty-Plus Reinfarction Study Group (1980) A double blind trial to assess long-term oral anticoagulant therapy in elderly patients after myocardial infarction. *Lancet* **ii**, 989–994.

Stein P.D. & Kantrowitz A. (1989) Antithrombotic therapy in mechanical and biological prosthetic heart valves and saphenous vein by-pass grafts. *Chest* **95**, 107S–117S.

Taberner D.A., Poller L., Burslem R.W. & Jones J.B. (1978) Oral anticoagulants controlled by the British Comparative Thromboplastin versus low-dose heparin prophylaxis of deep vein thrombosis. *British Medical Journal* **11**, 272.

Tomensen J. & Thomson J.M. (1985) Standardisation of the prothrombin time in blood coagulation and haemostasis. In Thomson J.M. (ed.) *Blood Coagulation and Haemostasis* 3rd edn, pp. 370–409. Churchill Livingstone, Edinburgh.

Turpie C.G., Gunstensen J., Hirsh J., Nelson H. & Gent M. (1988) Randomised comparison of two intensities of oral anticoagulant therapy after tissue heart valve replacement. *Lancet* **i**, 124–125.

Veterans Administration (1973) Anticoagulants in acute myocardial infarction. *Journal of the American Medical Association* **222**, 724–729.

9 Use and Monitoring of Heparin Therapy

Prepared by the
Haemostasis and Thrombosis Task Force

Properties of heparin

Heparin is a naturally occurring sulphated glycosaminoglycan produced by the mast cells of most species. It is extracted from bovine and porcine lungs or intestinal mucosa and virtually all heparin now used in the UK is mucosal. Heparin is prepared as a sterile solution of the sodium or calcium salt in water and is heat stable, but preparations generally have a shelf life of 3 years because of the possibility of bacterial contamination. Multidose vials normally contain a bacteriostatic preservative but a preservative-free product is also available. All commercial preparations are heterogeneous, consisting of mixtures of polysaccharides of molecular weights ranging from 5000 to 30 000, the heterogeneity occurring naturally during biosynthesis and not as a result of the extraction process. Activity is determined by biological assay against a reference standard. The two major pharmacopeial assays are the BP and the USP. The new BP assay (British Pharmacopoeia 1980, Addendum 1986) is based on the determination of the Activated Partial Thromboplastin Time (APTT) of citrated sheep plasma and is equivalent to the European Pharmacopeial Assay. The reference for the BP and most other assays is the International Standard, which defines the International Unit. Assays by the USP method, which measures the effect of heparin on the degree of coagulation of citrated sheep plasma, are generally referred to a separate USP standard, resulting in a USP unit, which differs from the International Unit by about 7–10%.

The anticoagulant action of heparin results from its binding to antithrombin III (AT III), thereby increasing the rate at which this inhibitor neutralizes the main serine protease enzymes of the coagulation cascade, i.e. Factors XIa, IXa, Xa and thrombin. The clinical effect of heparin depends upon the concentration of clotting factors, AT III, and many other heparin binding proteins, and the response of different individuals to the same dose varies enormously. Heparin also influences platelet function. Its action on the vascular endothelium by releasing lipase can clear lipaemic plasma.

Administration must be parenteral as oral heparin would be bound by gastric protein. It can be given subcutaneously through the adipose tissue of the abdominal wall and is well absorbed into the plasma from which it disappears relatively slowly. Intravenous administration gives a plasma half-life of 1–2 hours at the usual therapeutic doses. Metabolism occurs in the liver and a degraded form is excreted in the urine. Heparin does not cross the placental barrier or enter maternal milk.

Low molecular weight fractions of heparin (LMWH) have been prepared in the hope that they will be as effective as the standard form but cause less bleeding. There is also some evidence that the half-life of LMWH is longer than that of the unfractionated material. The results of controlled trials are beginning to appear (Thomas, 1986) and the potential for the prevention of deep vein thrombosis in patients undergoing elective hip surgery is of particular interest. LMWH may be available in the UK in the future.

The aim of therapy is to prevent the formation or local extension of thrombus and/or pulmonary embolism.

Therapeutic administration

Principal indications are deep vein thrombosis and pulmonary embolism. Less well substantiated indications include myocardial infarction and, in some cases, disseminated intravascular coagulation.

Principal contraindications are haemorrhagic states including thrombocytopenia, recent ophthalmic or neurosurgery, hypertension with diastolic pressure over 110 mmHg, peptic ulceration, oesophageal varices and known hypersensitivity to heparin.

Heparin can be given intravenously, by continuous infusion using a small infusion pump, or by intermittent subcutaneous injections into the anterior or anterolateral wall of the abdomen near the iliac crest or thigh using small volume syringes with small bore needles so that a precise dose can be delivered (Bentley *et al.*, 1980). The recommended concentration for subcutaneous administration is 25 000 IU/ml.

Dosage

INTRAVENOUS ADMINISTRATION

An intravenous loading dose of 5000 international units (IU) is followed by 1000–2000 IU/h (approx. 14–28 IU/kg/h) adjusted daily by laboratory monitoring.

SUBCUTANEOUS ADMINISTRATION

Full dose heparin can be given using a high concentration subcutaneous preparation at an initial dose of 10 000–20 000 units 12 hourly adjusted daily by laboratory monitoring. The clinical value of subcutaneous administration for treatment of pulmonary embolism is not yet established.

Laboratory monitoring

Daily laboratory monitoring is advised, preferably at the same time each day. The selected method is a matter for individual laboratories but should have a good linear relationship to graded concentrations of heparin added to plasma *in vitro* over a range of clinically relevant levels. The linearity of the dose response should be maintained up to 2.0 IU/ml. With an APTT technique, which is by far the most widely used method in the UK, the optimum therapeutic range is best defined by the individual laboratory and will vary, depending upon the APTT reagent in use. A broad guide is 1.5–2.5 times an average control reading. The calcium thrombin time is linear over a narrower range than the APTT but is not prolonged by oral anticoagulant drugs. The therapeutic range depends on the molarity of calcium chloride and the source and concentration of thrombin, and so must be determined by the individual laboratory (O'Shea *et al.*, 1971).

Adjustment of dose

If reduction of dosage is necessary, it is advisable to stop the infusion for about 30 to 60 minutes before reducing the dosage level; an increased dosage may require a bolus of 3000–5000 IU.

Duration of therapy

Parenteral therapy should continue until treatment is no longer required or until oral anticoagulants have achieved a therapeutic effect. This generally takes at least 3 days even if the prothrombin ratio falls within the appropriate therapeutic range earlier.

Prophylactic administration

Indications—to prevent deep vein thrombosis in certain patients at risk when undergoing a surgical procedure under general anaesthesia lasting over 30 minutes and requiring postoperative hospitalization.

In the context of general surgery high risk patients include those over the age of 40, those who are obese or have a malignancy or have had prior deep vein thrombosis or pulmonary embolism, or those undergoing large or complicated surgical procedures. Pregnant women and those requiring major orthopaedic surgery have special problems which are considered below. The prevention of deep venous thrombosis and pulmonary embolism in these and other situations has been the subject of a recent consensus development conference held by the US National Institutes of Health (Consensus Conference 1986).

Dosage

Pre-operative 2 hours—5000 IU subcutaneously.
Postoperative—5000 IU subcutaneously every 8–12 hours for seven days or until patient is mobile.

Pregnancy

To prevent thrombo-embolism in mothers with a history of deep vein thrombosis or pulmonary embolism, an initial recommended dosage is 10 000 IU 12 hourly or 7500 IU 8 hourly by self-administered subcutaneous injection. Periodic dose adjustment is desirable and an increase in dosage may be necessary in the last weeks of pregnancy. Warfarin may be substituted from 16 to 36 weeks maintaining the INR (BR) between 2.0 and 3.0. If heparin therapy is continued during labour its dosage should be carefully monitored, reduced at delivery and then resumed until anticoagulation is stopped or warfarin resumed. Detailed discussion is given by Letsky (1985).

The management of pregnant women with prosthetic heart valves is difficult and controversial. The problems are highlighted by Iturbe-Alessio *et al.* (1986). They found that low dose heparin (5000 units 12 hourly) was ineffective in preventing valve thrombosis while the incidence of embryopathy in patients receiving coumarin derivatives from the 6th to the 12th week of gestation was between 25 and 30%. A higher dose of heparin might have prevented valve thrombosis but there is no evidence that this approach would be successful. Women with artificial heart valves who wish to become pregnant therefore require careful counselling. In the event of pregnancy a reasonable policy would be to use heparin until 12–16 weeks followed by warfarin until 36 weeks and then revert to heparin as discussed above.

Laboratory monitoring

Generally, low dose subcutaneous heparin is not routinely monitored. A dose adjusted regime using APTT monitoring to maintain minimal prolongation of the test may be required in patients with malignant disease and for hip surgery or fractured femur both to ensure adequacy of dosage and safety (Hull *et al.*, 1982; Leyvraz *et al.*, 1983; Poller *et al.*, 1982). The value of heparin assays (Denson & Bonnar, 1973) in this group remains to be established but they may be useful where available.

Those who require heparin anticoagulation for pregnancy or prosthetic heart valves should be monitored with APTT levels being held at not less than 1.5 times an average control 2 hours following injection.

Complications

1 Haemorrhage is usually due to excess dosage or idiosyncrasy to conventional dosage. Withdrawal is usually sufficient but if bleeding continues, protamine sulphate antidote (approximately 1 mg protamine neutralizes 150 IU heparin) should be given slowly intravenously. Where possible, the dosage required should be calculated but should not exceed 40 mg in one injection. Epidural anaesthesia is contraindicated when heparin is being used.
2 Thrombocytopenia.
3 Alopecia.
4 Local skin necrosis from hypersensitivity.
5 Osteoporosis. This has been a problem in patients maintained on long term therapy.
6 Anaphylactic shock.
7 Abortion.

References

Bentley P.G., Kakkar V.V., Scully M.F., MacGregor I.R., Webb P., Chan P. & Jones N. (1980) An objective study of alternative methods of heparin administration. *Thrombosis Research* **18**, 177–187.

Consensus Conference—Prevention of venous thrombosis and pulmonary embolism (1986) *Journal of the American Medical Association*, **245** 744–749.

Denson K.W.E. & Bonnar J. (1973) The measurement of heparin. A method based on the potentiation of anti-factor Xa. *Thrombosis et Diathesis Haemorrhagica* **30**, 471–479.

Hull R., Delmore T., Carter C., Hirsh J., Genton E., Gent M., Turpie G. & McLaughlin D. (1982) Adjusted subcutaneous heparin versus warfarin sodium in the long term treatment of venous thrombosis. *New England Journal of Medicine* **306**, 189–194.

Iturbe-Alessio I., del Carmen Fonseca M., Mutchinik O., Santos M.A., Zajarias A. & Salazar E. (1986) Risks of anticoagulant therapy in pregnant women with artificial heart valves. *New England Journal of Medicine* **315**, 1390–1393.

Letsky E.A., (1985) *Coagulation Problems During Pregnancy.* Churchill Livingstone, Edinburgh.

Leyvraz P.F., Richard J., Bachmann F., van Melle G., Treyvaud J-M., Livio J-J. & Candardjis G. (1983) Adjusted versus fixed-dose subcutaneous heparin in the prevention of deep-vein thrombosis after total hip replacement. *New England Journal of Medicine* **309**, 954–958.

Poller L., Taberner D.A., Sandilands D.G. & Galasko C.S.B. (1982) An evaluation of APTT monitoring of low-dose heparin dosage in hip surgery. *Thrombosis and Haemostasis* **47**, 50–53.

O'Shea M.J., Flute P.T. & Pannell G.M. (1971) Laboratory control of heparin therapy. *Journal of Clinical Pathology* **24**, 542–546.

Thomas D.P. (1986) Current status of low molecular weight heparin. *Thrombosis and Haemostasis* **56**, 241–242.

10 Platelet Function Testing

Prepared by the
Haemostasis and Thrombosis Task Force

Following a questionnaire from the Haemostasis and Thrombosis Task Force of the British Society for Haematology in 1985, there was obviously considerable variability and confusion as to how haematologists in the UK investigated platelet function. This chapter outlines a standardized approach which could be followed by most routine laboratories for the investigation of bleeding disorders. Platelet release studies are included for interest; these are not recommended for routine laboratories. Platelet function studies used specifically to investigate thrombotic disorders or an assumed hypercoaguable state will not be discussed in these guidelines. Tests which are primarily of a research nature or are in use only at a highly specialized referral unit are also not discussed. It is essential to have a working knowledge of platelet physiology so that the relevant platelet function tests can be performed in an orderly sequence and interpreted correctly (Yardumian *et al.*, 1986; Vermylen *et al.*, 1983). For this reason we have supplied some basic details on platelet biochemistry and structure.

The bleeding time

Background

When investigating patients suspected of having a bleeding disorder, it is essential to obtain a detailed clinical history before embarking on tests of haemostatic function.

The peripheral platelet count, blood film examination, and the skin bleeding time are the first line basic laboratory tests of platelet function. If these tests are within normal limits it is unlikely that a clinically important platelet defect is responsible for excessive clinical bleeding.

A drug history is particularly important, and as far as possible the use of drugs should be avoided when platelet function is assessed. This applies particularly topatients with congenital platelet disorders. In acquired bleeding states the drugs

Reprinted with permission from the *Journal of Clinical Pathology*, 1988, **41**, 1322–1330.

that patients are receiving may themselves be directly responsible for the haemostatic defect. When this is suspected platelet function should be assessed when the patient is both off and on the drug. Recent aspirin ingestion is of particular importance as a single dose may exert its effect for up to 10 days. Other drugs which affect the bleeding time include non-steroidal anti-inflammatory agents, ticlopidine, heparin, penicillin (in high doses) and the antibiotics carbenicillin and ticarcillin (Table 10.1).

The bleeding time is arguably the most useful test of platelet function in that it provides clinically relevant information about the contribution of platelets to primary haemostasis.

Table 10.1 Drugs which affect platelet function

Membrane stabilizing agents
α-antagonists
β-blockers
Local anaesthetics (procaine)
Antihistamines
Tricyclic antidepressants
Frusemide
Agents which affect prostanoid synthesis
Aspirin and proprietary preparations containing acetylsalicylic acid
Non-steroid anti-inflammatory
Corticosteroids
Antibiotics
Penicillins
Cephalosporins
β-lactam derivatives
Agents which increase cyclic adenosine monophosphatase concentrations
Dipyridamole
Aminophylline
Prostanoids
Others
Heparin
Dextrans
Ethanol
Phenothiazine
Clofibrate
Papaverine
Foodstuffs
Alcohol
Garlic
Certain Chinese foods

How long it takes for bleeding to stop after a skin incision is largely influenced by rapid accumulation of metabolically active platelets at the site of the wound and the formation of a haemostatically effective platelet plug. The bleeding time reflects this process and if it is performed in a standardized manner is sensitive to changes in platelet function and platelet number.

Several attempts have been made to improve the sensitivity and reproducibility of the bleeding time since its introduction in 1910 by Duke. In the original method the ear lobe was punctured by a needle. Later, between 1935 and 1941, Ivy described a method which consisted of three puncture wounds in the forearm. Some improvement in sensitivity was achieved by the application of a sphygmomanometer cuff, inflated to 40 mm Hg pressure, at a site proximal to the puncture wounds.

Recently, further modifications of the bleeding time have resulted in a test that is both sensitive and reproducible. In 1958 Borchgrevink and Waaler recommended the use of incisions of predetermined length and depth rather than puncture wounds. Additional refinements were described by Mielke in 1969 and more recently a disposable spring loaded device (Simplate II, General Diagnostics) has been developed which produces incisions 5 mm long and 1 mm deep and gives reliable and reproducible results (Mielke, 1982).

Methodology

A recent survey of UK laboratories studied striking differences in reported bleeding times of normal subjects (Poller *et al.*, 1984). These differences were even apparent among laboratories using template bleeding times. These observations emphasise the necessity for strict laboratory control, and it is therefore strongly recommended that for any given method individual laboratories should establish their own range of normal values. The result may be influenced by the choice of operator and this also should be borne in mind when establishing the normal range.

For the reasons outlined above, the template bleeding time is the method of choice (Greaves & Preston, 1985). After a sphygmomanometer cuff, inflated to 40 mmHg pressure, has been applied, incisions are made over the lateral aspect of the anterior surface of the forearm, care being taken to avoid superficial veins. After 30 seconds the blood issuing from the wound is gently blotted with filter paper. The wound edge is not touched. Blotting is continued at 30 second intervals until the blood no longer stains the filter paper. This represents the bleeding time end point.

Duplicate incisions are recommended unless it can be shown that reliable results can be achieved by a single incision.

Factors influencing the bleeding time

The bleeding time is influenced by several factors including age, sex, skin temperature, haematocrit, venostasis and the site and direction of the incision. The most important variables are those which relate to methodological detail.

The bleeding time is longer when the incision is made on the lateral, as opposed to the medial aspect of the forearm, and a transverse incision produces a longer bleeding time than does one which is performed longitudinally. Many workers recommend a longitudinal technique as scarring is a potential problem with transverse incisions. The use of a 'butterfly' dressing to approximate the wound edges may also minimize the risk of scarring.

When performed without venostasis pronounced variation of the bleeding time can occur. The use of a sphygmomanometer cuff, inflated to 40 mmHg pressure, produces longer bleeding times and reduces the degree of variability.

Several workers have shown that there is a significant difference in bleeding times between males and females, with longer times being recorded in females. Although cold is known to prolong the bleeding time it is probably important only when the skin temperature falls below 25 °C.

The platelet count also influences the bleeding time; as this falls below $80–100 \times 10^9$/l the bleeding time becomes progressively prolonged. In most patients with thrombocytopenia a bleeding time is therefore unnecessary. In a proportion, however, the bleeding time may be of clinical value in that it provides information about platelet reactivity. An example is disseminated intravascular coagulation where an acquired storage pool disorder may accompany thrombocytopenia. On these occasions the bleeding time will be disproportionately prolonged relative to the platelet count.

In normal neonates and children the bleeding time may be longer than that of adults. Although the establishment of a normal range in these groups is highly desirable, this may be precluded on ethical grounds. For departments where this applies, useful experience can be obtained by performing the technique in a standardized manner but results should be interpreted with appropriate caution.

If the bleeding time suggests a platelet functional disorder, or when there is a high degree of clinical suspicion despite a normal bleeding time, further tests should be planned in a systematic way. Drugs and certain dietary practices (Table 10.1) are the most common cause of platelet dysfunction (Packham & Mustard, 1977) and ideally patients should refrain from taking drugs with known antiplatelet effects for seven to 10 days before blood sampling for more specific function investigation. If there is any doubt about a particular drug the bleeding time should be repeated if possible 2 weeks after stopping that drug. Causes of a prolonged bleeding time are summarized in Table 10.2. In most instances these relate to changed platelet reactivity. Special attention should be paid to the possibility of von Willebrand's disease and its many variants.

Table 10.2 Causes of a prolonged skin bleeding time

Thrombocytopenia	Congenital qualitative platelet disorders	Congenital deficiency of coagulation factors	Hereditary connective tissue disorders	Acquired states
Due to marrow failure	Bernard–Soulier syndrome	von Willebrand's disease	Ehlers–Danlos syndrome (Type III)	Liver failure
Due to platelet consumption or destruction	Glanzmann's thrombasthenia	Afibrinogenaemia		Uraemia
	Store pool disease and syndrome	Factor V deficiency	Osteogenesis imperfecta	Dysproteinaemia
	Gray platelet syndrome			Myeloproliferative disease
	Cyclo-oxygenase deficiency			Acquired storage pool disease
	Thromboxane synthase deficiency			Drugs
	Other unclassified			Diet
				Severe anaemia
				Polycythaemia (secondary)

Tests of platelet adhesion

The most widely adopted diagnostic adhesion test measures platelet retention after a single passage of whole blood through a glass bead column. Attempts to standardize this test have used glass beads of a constant size packed in a tube of fixed diameter and length (which are commercially available) with a steady infusion rate of non-anticoagulated whole blood directly from an arm vein, using an evacuated system. The percentage platelet retention in the column is calculated from a pre- and post-column infusion platelet count. Despite all these precautions the results are extremely variable and decreased glass bead retention of platelets is not only found in platelet adhesion defects. It has subsequently been shown that retention also depends on plasma von Willebrand factor (factor VIII: WF) activity, fibrinogen coating the glass bead surface, and on platelet aggregation which is promoted by local release of adenosine diphosphate (ADP) from haemolyzed red cells in the column. These tests are therefore not generally recommended as a routine platelet function test.

Platelet aggregation

Studies of platelet aggregation are indicated in anyone suspected of having a platelet function defect, particularly in patients with a prolonged or borderline bleeding time test. These tests are routinely performed on platelet rich plasma. Recently techniques using whole blood have been developed (Lumley & Humphrey, 1981; Mackie *et al.*, 1984) but because of their limitations for routine use and difficulties in interpretation they will not be further discussed here.

Turbidometric method

PRINCIPLE

Blood is centrifuged gently to obtain platelet rich plasma, which is stirred in a cuvette at 37°C between a light source and a photocell. When an agonist is added, the platelets aggregate and absorb less light so that transmission increases and is detected by movement of a pen on the chart recorder. The addition of different agonists at a range of concentrations allows certain aggregation defects to be detected.

BIOCHEMICAL BASIS

Reagents such as collagen, thrombin, and ADP bind to specific platelet membrane receptors, activating platelets and triggering a series of reactions which can culminate in shape change, granule release, and aggregation. Whether any or all of these responses occur depends on the normal function of the platelet, the concentrations of certain inhibitory substances, and the concentration of the agonist used.

There are thought to be three basic pathways of platelet aggregation all of which are interlinked: ADP causes a chain of events involving phosphatidyl inositol metabolism, leading to the exposure of fibrinogen binding sites on the membrane and aggregation. Low concentrations of collagen cause platelet aggregation through a pathway predominantly dependent on prostaglandin biosynthesis. This induces arachidonic acid mobilization from the membrane, followed by conversion to thromboxane A_2, which is a potent stimulator of aggregation, causing ADP release and calcium flux. Higher concentrations of collagen will also activate platelets by prostaglandin independent mechanisms. Similar considerations apply to low and high concentrations of thrombin. Serotonin and adrenaline act synergistically with other reagents. The relation of *in vitro* platelet aggregation in plasma to physiological responses must be considered carefully as the low extracellular calcium ion concentrations generate artefacts such as the release reactions to ADP and adrenaline, which do not occur if blood is collected into the thrombin inhibitor hirudin, instead of citrate.

TEST SAMPLES

Nine volumes of blood are added to one volume of trisodium citrate (0.109 M) and citrated blood is then centrifuged at 170 *g* (800–1000 rpm in a bench centrifuge), for 10 minutes at room temperature to prepare platelet rich plasma. This must be removed and stored at room temperature in a capped tube. All handling should be kept to a minimum and be done with plastic pipettes and tubes.

The residual blood must then be centrifuged at 2700 *g* (about 3500 rpm) for 15 minutes and the resulting platelet poor plasma collected.

REAGENTS

1 ADP (Sigma Grade III): 10 mM solution in saline, stored in aliquots at −20°C.
2 Collagen (Hormon-Chemie, München): 1 mg/ml stored at 4°C.
3 Adrenaline (Sigma): 1 mg/ml (5.5 mM) store at −20°C.
4 Arachidonate (Sigma): 20 mM solution in distilled water, store at −20°C.
5 Thrombin (Parke-Davis, Bovine): 50 u/ml solution in saline, at −20°C.
6 Endoperoxide Analogue U46619 (Upjohn Ltd): dissolve phial contents in a small quantity of ethanol and dilute to 25 μg/ml with saline, store at −20°C in aliquots.
7 Calcium Ionophore A23187, Ca^{2+} + Mg^{2+} salt (Sigma): 500 μ/ml (1 mM) in ethanol at −20°C.
8 Ristocetin (Lundbeck): 12.5 mg/ml in saline, store at −20°C.
9 Porcine FVIII Complex/Bovine Fibrinogen (Diagnostic Reagents Ltd), reconstitute according to manufacturer.

EQUIPMENT

1 Optical aggregometer—the method described is for an aggregometer, which does not have an autobaseline facility, fitted with cuvettes for 250–500 μl.
2 Chart recorder.
3 Glass cuvettes.
4 Stir bars.
5 Equipment for platelet counting.

PREPARATION OF SAMPLES AND REAGENTS

Platelet rich plasma is diluted with autologous platelet poor plasma to give a final platelet count of 200×10^9/l.

ADP—prepare 100, 50, 25, 10, and 5 μM solutions in saline on ice.

Collagen—prepare 40 and 10 μg/ml solutions in buffer (Hormon-Chemie) on ice.

Ristocetin—thaw stock and keep on ice. Dilute as necessary in saline.

Adrenaline—prepare 100, 50, and 10 μM solutions in saline on ice.

Arachidonate—dilute stock solution with an equal volume of distilled water on ice.

Thrombin—dilute in saline to 1 and 5 μ/ml on ice.

Calcium Ionophore A23187—dilute in saline to give 5 and 100 μg/ml solutions, store on ice.

Porcine Factor VIII—dilute to 20 u/ml at room temperature.

METHOD

1 Allow aggregometer to warm at 37°C and set stirrer speed to 900 rpm.
2 Set chart recorder to 10 mV and 3 cm/minute.
3 Platelet poor plasma (300 μl) is placed in one cuvette and 270 μl platelet rich plasma with a stir bar in another; these are used to calibrate the aggregometer signal on the chart recorder to 10% and 95% settings, using the output and zero controls, respectively (see manufacturer's instructions).
4 Undiluted platelet rich plasma (270 μl) is placed in a cuvette in the aggregometer and stirred for 15 minutes to check for spontaneous aggregation (pen deflection > 20% of chart).
5 If spontaneous aggregation is present dilute the platelet rich plasma in platelet poor plasma and repeat the test until a dilution is found where spontaneous aggregation disappears. If this point is found at or above a platelet count of 200×10^9/l, aggregation tests may proceed.
6 Place 270 μl dilute platelet rich plasma in a cuvette and warm until a steady baseline is obtained.
7 Add 30 μl of aggregating reagent (agonist) and record response.
8 Continue with other agonists at the final concentration range indicated (Table 10.3).

The three agonists listed in Table 10.3 should be initially used routinely over the final concentration ranges stated. Only if defective aggregation responses are obtained should one proceed with the agents listed.

EXPRESSION AND REPORTING OF RESULTS

Subjective assessment of aggregation responses by a trained eye is usually sufficient for clinical interpretations. Typical traces obtained with some commonly used aggregating agents are shown in Figure 10.1. Quantitation of the

Table 10.3 Agonists for platelet aggregation studies

Agents routinely used in screening tests	Final concentrations usually used
ADP	0·5–10·0 μM
Collagen	1·0–4·0 μg/ml†
*Ristocetin	0·5–1·2 mg/ml
Other agents in routine use	
Adrenaline	1·0–10·0 μM
Thrombin	0·1–0·5 u/ml
Arachidonic acid	1·0–2·0 μ/M

* Agents causing platelet agglutination rather than true aggregation.
† This varies according to species and tissue source of collagen. The manufacturer's instructions should be followed.

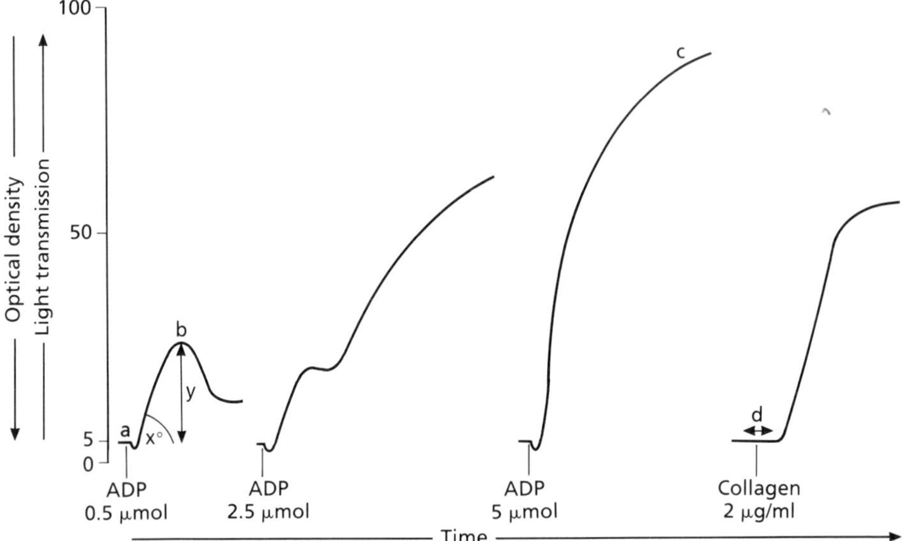

Fig. 10.1 Typical traces obtained during platelet-rich plasma aggregation: a = shape change; b = primary wave aggregation; c = secondary wave aggregation; x° = angle of ascent of aggregation trace; y = height of aggregation trace; d = lag phase.

aggregation response may be made by measuring the lag phase (*d*) (with collagen only) the angle (*x*) of the initial aggregation slope, and the maximum height (*y*) of the response after a standard time (usually 3 minutes). Alternatively, threshold concentrations may be determined by starting with a very low dose of an aggregating agent and progressively adding higher concentrations of the agonist until a response is obtained. Similarly, an EC_{50} (50% of effective concentration) value can be obtained by finding the dose of aggregating reagent which causes 50% of the maximum response; this is usually found by drawing a dose-response curve for a number of concentrations of agonist.

TECHNICAL COMMENTS

1 The volumes of platelet rich plasma used will depend on the aggregometer and cuvettes used. The smaller the cuvette, the more responses that can be obtained with a given volume of platelet rich plasma, but the poorer the optical quality (due to a shorter lightpath) and the more likely the influence of factors such as debris or air bubbles.

2 Care should be taken to exclude red cells and granulocytes from platelet rich plasma as these will interfere with the light transmittance and cause reduced response heights which can be mistaken for abnormal aggregation. In diseases such as thalassaemia, where there may be red cell fragments and membranes, these may be removed by further centrifugation of platelet rich plasma at 150 *g* for 2 minutes, or after settling has occurred.

3 If cryoglobulins are present they may cause changes in transmittance like spontaneous aggregation. Warming the platelet rich plasma to 37°C for 5 minutes allows aggregation to be performed in the normal way.

4 Lipaemic plasma may cause problems in adjusting the aggregometer and the responses may be compressed owing to the small difference in transmitted light between platelet rich plasma and platelet poor plasma. Care should be taken in the interpretation of results from such samples.

5 The aggregometer must be adjusted with platelet rich plasma at the platelet count that will be used in the test, as this will affect optical density—for example, when changing from spontaneous aggregation to responses to agonists.

6 Aggregation should be performed within 2 hours. If longer delays cannot be avoided it is best to store the platelet rich plasma under 5% carbon dioxide, or if this is not available, to leave the smallest possible air gap over the platelet rich plasma and cap the tube.

7 Lumi-aggregometers are also available; these measure ATP release simultaneously with aggregation. This is possible using a firefly extract known as luciferase, which emits energy in the form of luminescence when ATP is available as a substrate; the latter can be detected if a luminescence detector is fitted to the aggregometer.

8 Ristocetin concentrations above 1.4 mg/ml may cause non-specific protein precipitation which can be mistaken for agglutination. Absent aggregation induced by ristocetin may occur in patients of Afro-Caribbean racial origin and is not associated with a bleeding diathesis.

INTERPRETATION

Patterns of typical abnormal aggregation responses are shown in Table 10.4.

For a more detailed discussion of aggregation agonist responses and

Table 10.4 Patterns of abnormal aggregation

Disorder	ADP	Collagen	Ristocetin (1.2 mg/ml)	Ristocetin (0.5 mg/ml)	Arachidonic acid	Endoperoxide analogue	A23187	Porcine VIII	Confirmatory tests
vW disease (type I and IIA)	N	N	A/R/N	A	N	N	N	N	Factor VIII studies
vW disease (type IIB)	N	N	N	H	N	N	N	N	Factor VIII studies
Bernard–Soulier syndrome	N	N	A	A	N	N	N	A	Not required
Glanzmann's thrombasthenia	A	A	N	A	A	A	—	P	Not required
Storage pool disease	P/N	R/N	P/N	A	R/N	R/N	R/N	P/N	Nucleotides 5-HT release studies
Membrane receptor defect	R/N	R	R/N	A	N	N	N	N	
Cyclo-oxygenase deficiency	R/N	R	N	A	R	N	N	N	

N–Normal response; A–Absent response; R–Reduced response; H–Heightened increased response; P–Primary wave only.

congenital and acquired defects of platelet function, the following reviews are useful: Yardumian *et al.* (1986), Greaves and Preston (1985), Hardisty (1983), Raio and Walsh (1983).

The release reaction and platelet adenine nucleotide measurement

The platelet release reaction is characterized by secretion of the constituents of the three types of platelet storage granule. These comprise dense bodies, α granules, and lysosomes.

Dense bodies are the storage site for calcium, serotonin, and the non-metabolic pool of adenine nucleotides. As they are osmiophilic and absorb electrons when unstained they appear as dense intraplatelet inclusions on transmission electron microscopy.

Alpha granules contain several platelet specific proteins, such as platelet factor 4 and β-thromboglobulin, and certain coagulation factors. The stimulus to release α granule contents is often less than that for dense body release and increased plasma concentrations of the aforementioned platelet specific proteins may be interpreted as evidence of platelet activation.

In the investigation of patients with bleeding disorders the release mechanism is usually assessed by determination of the total platelet content of ADP and adenosine triphosphate (ATP), and the release of ATP or 5-hydroxytryptamine or both, from the dense bodies.

There are two separate nucleotide pools within the platelet, with 60% being stored in the dense granules. The remainder constitute the metabolic pool of adenine nucleotides. There are pronounced differences in the relative concentrations of ADP and ATP within the two pools. In the metabolic pool the ATP : ADP ratio is 8 : 1; in the dense granules the ratio is 2 : 3. The nucleotide exchange between the pools is slow. Thus in storage pool defects where there is reduction or absence of dense bodies and their associated nucleotides the ratio of total platelet ATP to total platelet ADP increases.

There are various methods for determining total platelet nucleotides (Greaves & Preston, 1985). In routine clinical practice assays based on firefly bioluminescence techniques are increasingly being used. The firefly enzyme luciferase produces light proportional to the concentration of ATP and this is measured with a luminometer. Although ADP cannot be measured directly by this method, it is possible to perform an indirect assay by converting the available ADP to ATP.

Firefly bioluminescence techniques are also of value in assessing platelet release. This has been facilitated by the recent introduction of an aggregometer which also incorporates a luminometer. The system therefore permits simultaneous monitoring of platelet aggregation and platelet release of ATP.

High performance liquid chromatography is a more sensitive method for measuring platelet adenine nucleotides but it is not generally available in routine haematology departments.

5-hydroxytryptamine (5-HT) is readily taken up by platelets and stored in the dense bodies. Determination of the uptake and release of 5-HT by platelets is a convenient method of assessing platelet secretion. In this system thrombin or some other agonist is used to induce platelet secretion and the proportion of incorporated radioactivity released from the platelets determined. Additional information can also be obtained by measuring the proportion of radioactivity that 'leaks' from unstimulated platelets. Normally this does not occur but it may be detectable in storage pool disorders.

Before investigating platelet release it is important for each laboratory to establish its own normal range with respect to the agonist and also to the concentration used. Thrombin induces the release of 70–90% total radioactivity while that induced by collagen is somewhat less—20–60%. When using collagen it is important to use the same reagent throughout as the result is influenced by the type of collagen used.

ATP release: luciferin-luciferase method

Principle

When a platelet aggregating agent is added to platelet rich plasma in the presence of luciferin-luciferase, the ATP released during platelet aggregation will react with the luciferin in a light-emitting reaction:

$$\text{ATP} + \text{luciferin} \xrightarrow[\text{luciferase}]{\text{Mg}^{2+}} \text{adenyl luciferin}$$

The light released is measured and recorded by the lumiaggregometer.

REAGENTS

Luciferin-luciferase 40 mg/ml (Sigma)
ATP standard 100 μm (Sigma)
Arachidonic acid, sodium salt 15 μm (BioData)
Collagen 40 μg/ml (Hormon-Chemie, Munich)

METHOD

1 Take 18 ml blood into 2 ml 0.19 M sodium citrate in a plastic container, using a 19 gauge needle and minimum stasis.
2 Prepare platelet rich plasma as for platelet aggregation studies.
3 Prepare platelet poor plasma by centrifuging the remainder of the sample for 10 minutes at 2000 *g*.
4 Adjust platelet rich plasma count to 200×10^9/l with platelet poor plasma.
5 Using 500 μl platelet poor plasma and 450 μl platelet rich plasma, add the appropriate amount of freshly prepared luciferin-luciferase (25 μl for collagen, 50 μl for arachidonate) to the platelet rich plasma in a cuvette in the aggregometer and warm for 1 minute.
6 Add 50 μl of the appropriate agonist.
7 Observe the aggregation and record the luminescence in terms of peak height.
8 When the aggregation is complete add 20 μl (2 nmol) of ATP standard and record the peak height. Ideally the luminescence peak height should fall between that of the two standards, so if the luminescence peak is low use less standard, such as 10 μl and 15 μl.
9 Plot the standard concentrations as nmol against peak heights and read off the release peak obtained with each agonist.

CALCULATION

ATP release is expressed in terms of nmol/10^8 platelets:

$$\text{ATP release} = \frac{\text{nmol ATP released}}{\text{No. of platelets} \times 10^8 \times 0.45}$$

(0.45 is the volume of platelet rich plasma in the cuvette in ml.)

INTERPRETATION

Laboratories should establish their own normal ranges. Reduced ATP release indicates a platelet release defect.

Radiolabelled 5-hydroxytryptamine (serotonin) uptake and release

Principle

Serotonin is present in the dense granules of platelets and is released when the platelets aggregate. Platelets will also actively take up serotonin from solution.

Platelets are incubated with radiolabelled serotonin. The amount taken up by platelet dense bodies is measured as the difference between the total added radioactivity and the activity remaining in the incubation solution after the platelets are removed by centrifugation. Imipramine is added to prevent further uptake.

The platelets are aggregated with collagen or thrombin, or both and the amount of serotonin released measured. The amount of serotonin leaking out of the platelets is also determined.

REAGENTS

1 Imipramine hydrochloride: 31.5 mg in 5 ml distilled water, prepared fresh.
2 Thrombin 500 U/ml.
3 Collagen 40 μg/ml: make up as for platelet aggregation.
4 Stock ^{14}C-5-HT: prepare 0.5 ml volumes containing 1.258 μCi ^{14}C-5-HT.
5 Streptokinase 25 000 U/ml store at − 80°C.

PROCEDURE

1 Prepare platelet rich plasma from citrated blood, as for platelet aggregation studies. Adjust the platelet count to 200×10^9/l using platelet poor plasma. A control from a healthy donor should be studied concurrently.
2 Add 4.5 ml of platelet rich plasma to a 0.5 ml aliquot of ^{14}C-5-HT. Mix gently and incubate at 37°C in a water bath. Start the stopwatch.
3 Remove 0.5 ml for measurement of total counts. Transfer duplicate 100 μl aliquots to scintillation phials for counting (phials 1 and 2).
4 At 30 minutes, 60 minutes, and 90 minutes, remove 0.5 ml for measurement of uptake. Centrifuge to prepare platelet free plasma (an Eppendorf centrifuge is suitable) and transfer 100 μl aliquots of supernatant to scintillation phials (phials 3 and 4, 5 and 6, 7 and 8).
5 At 90 minutes add 3 μl of imipramine solution (final concentration 2×10^{-5}M). At 120 minutes remove 0.5 ml. Centrifuge as above and transfer 100 μl aliquots for counting. This represents 'leakage' (phials 9 and 10).
6 Remove 1 ml and incubate at room temperature on a rotary mixer, with 10 μl thrombin 500 μ/ml and 10 μl streptokinase 2500 U/ml, for about 10 minutes. Centrifuge and transfer 100 μl aliquots of supernatant for counting. This represents 'release to thrombin' (phials 11 and 12).
7 Remove 300 μl and transfer to an aggregometer cuvette with stirrer bar. Add 30 μl collagen to give a final concentration of 4 μg/ml and incubate in an

aggregometer for 5 minutes at 37°C. Centrifuge and transfer 100 μl aliquots for counting. This represents 'release to collagen' (phials 13 and 14).

CALCULATION

Calculate:

1 Mean of each replicate count.

2 Mean of each duplicate phial.

3 $\%\ \text{Uptake} = \dfrac{\text{Total counts} - \text{uptake counts}}{\text{Total counts}} \times 100$

Calculate uptake at T30, T60 and T90.

4 $\%\ \text{Leakage} = \dfrac{\text{Leakage counts} - \text{T90 uptake counts}}{\text{Total counts} - \text{T90 uptake counts}} \times 100$

5 $\%\ \text{Release} = \dfrac{\text{Release counts} - \text{leakage counts}}{\text{Total counts} - \text{leakage counts}} \times 100$

Calculate release to collagen and to thrombin.

INTERPRETATION OF RESULTS

For each agonist, normal ranges should be established for 5-HT uptake and release. Using the above procedure, thrombin is a more potent stimulus to 5-HT release than collagen (70–90% release compared with 20–60%, respectively), but in respect of collagen the result is influenced by the type used. Reduced 5-HT release indicates a platelet release defect. Normally, the 'leakage' of 5-HT from platelets is 0–8%. Increased values suggest a storage pool defect.

Conclusions

These guidelines outline the routine methodology which should be available for the initial investigation of a patient with a presumed haemorrhagic platelet defect. Platelet release studies are included for interest and are not recommended for routine laboratories.

Because of the importance of platelet aggregation by the standard turbidometric technique, this has been described in greater practical detail as it is with this widely available laboratory test that a great deal of confusion has arisen. For further details the reader is referred to two more detailed articles (Yardumian *et al.*, 1986; Greaves & Preston, 1985) by members of this Task Force. To help haematologists identify congenital disorders we enclose minimal diagnostic criteria (see Appendix).

Appendix: Congenital platelet disorders: minimal diagnostic criteria

GLANZMANN'S THROMBASTHENIA

1 Absent aggregation responses to ADP.
2 Primary agglutination response to ristocetin.

BERNARD–SOULIER SYNDROME

1 Large platelets on peripheral blood film.
2 Absent ristocetin-induced platelet agglutination not corrected by normal plasma (or cryoprecipitate).

PLATELET RELEASE DEFECTS

Impaired secondary aggregatory response to ADP. In some instances these responses are normal (Nieuwenhuis *et al.*, 1987). This group can be further categorized by the demonstration of additional features.
1 Storage pool disorders: increased platelet ATP:ADP ratio with reduced platelet ADP concentration.
2 Defect of arachidonic acid peroxidation—for example, cyclo-oxygenase deficiency, thromboxane synthetase deficiency.
  (a) Impaired arachidonate-induced platelet aggregation with normal primary aggregatory responses to ADP.
  (b) Reduced arachidonate-induced platelet thromboxane production.
3 Presumed abnormalities of Ca^{2+} mobilization: impaired aggregation responses to calcium ionophore (A23187).

GRAY PLATELET SYNDROME

1 Morphological abnormalities on peripheral blood film (typically, absence of azurophilic granules).
2 Evidence of reduced α granule platelet specific peptides (PF_4 and βTG).

FAMILIAL PLATELET

1 Giant platelet syndromes (excluding Bernard–Soulier)
  (a) Large platelets on blood film
  (b) Exclusion of Bernard–Soulier syndrome.
2 Congenital thrombocytopenia with normal platelet morphology.

PLATELET-TYPE ('PSEUDO') VON WILLEBRAND'S DISEASE

1 Features suggesting type 11A von Willebrand's disease.

2 Enhanced agglutination with ristocetin or agglutination by cryoprecipitate in the absence of ristocetin.

References

Greaves M. & Preston F.E. (1985) The laboratory investigation of acquired and congenital platelet disorders. In Thomson J.M. (ed.) *Blood Coagulation and Haemostasis: A Practical Guide* 3rd edn, pp. 56–134. Churchill Livingstone, Edinburgh.

Hardisty R.M. (1983) Hereditary disorders of platelet function. *Journal of Clinical Pathology* **12**, 153–174.

Lumley P. & Humphrey P.P.A. (1981) A method for quantitating platelet aggregation and analysing drug receptor interfon platelets in whole blood *in vitro*. *Journal of Pharmacological Methods* **6**, 153–166.

Mackie I.J., Jones R. & Machin S.J. (1984) Platelet impedance aggregation in whole blood and its inhibition by antiplatelet drugs. *Journal of Clinical Pathology* **37**, 874–878.

Mielke C.H. (1982) Measurement of the bleeding time. *Thrombosis and Haemostasis* **52**, 210–211.

Nieuwenhuis H.K., Akkerman J.N. & Sixma J.J. (1987) Patients with a prolonged bleeding time and normal aggregation tests may have storage pool deficiency. *Blood* **70**, 620–623.

Packham M.A. & Mustard J.F. (1977) Clinical pharmacology of platelets. *Blood* 555–567.

Poller L., Thomson J.M. & Tomensen J.A. (1984) The bleeding time: current practice in the UK. *Clinical and Laboratory Haematology* **6**, 369–373.

Raio A.K. & Walsh P.N. (1983) Acquired qualitative platelet disorders. *Clinics in Haematology* **12**, 201–238.

Vermylen J., Badenhorst P.N., Deckmyn H. & Arnout J. (1983) Normal mechanisms of platelet function. *Clinics in Haematology* **12**, 107–152.

Yardumian D.A., Mackie I.J. & Machin S.J. (1986) Laboratory investigation of platelet function: a review of methodology. *Journal of Clinical Pathology* **39**, 701–712.

11 The Investigation and Management of Thrombophilia

Prepared by the
Haemostasis and Thrombosis Task Force

Definition

After much discussion, the Haemostasis and Thrombosis Task Force of the British Society for Haematology has agreed that the term *thrombophilia* be used to describe 'the familial or acquired disorders of the haemostatic mechanism which are likely to predispose to thrombosis'.

Thrombosis becomes more common as age increases and its occurrence is frequently associated with so-called 'risk factors' such as trauma (accidental or surgical), pregnancy, malignant disease or immobilization. Thrombosis, however, may develop at a younger age and sometimes in the absence of an easily identifiable 'risk factor', apparently spontaneously. Recently it has been increasingly recognized that patients who have defects or abnormalities which alter the physiological haemostatic balance in favour of fibrin formation or persistence are at increased risk of clinical thrombosis. These patients may be considered to have thrombophilia. It must however be realized that many patients with laboratory evidence of a thrombophilic abnormality remain clinically asymptomatic.

In inherited thrombophilia, thromboses are most commonly venous but in some thrombophilic disorders, particularly in acquired disorders, the risk of arterial thrombosis is also increased.

Mechanisms of thrombosis

Over the past 10 years it has become increasingly evident that the so-called thrombo-haemorrhagic balance is maintained by complicated interactions between the coagulation system, the fibrinolytic system, platelets and the vessel wall.

It is hypothesized that small amounts of activated factor X and activated factor V are continuously generated within the vascular system (Bauer & Rosenberg, 1987). These activated coagulation components bind to specific platelet receptors to form prothrombinase complex and to produce small amounts of thrombin.

Natural anticoagulants, for example antithrombin III (ATIII) and the Protein C/Protein S (PC/PS) system oppose this generation of thrombin.

Activation of platelets disrupts platelet membrane phospholipids, exposing a negatively charged exterior surface which, in the presence of calcium ions, offers a favourable binding locale for prothrombin. Prothrombin is therefore brought into close contact with prothrombinase complex on the platelet surface. Significant amounts of thrombin can thus be generated which may overwhelm the natural anticoagulant mechanisms and allow thrombin cleavage of fibrinogen.

Plasmin digests fibrin producing soluble cleavage products. The generation of plasmin is limited by the availability of plasminogen and regulated by mechanisms which govern the release of plasminogen activators and fibrinolytic inhibitors from cellular sites. It is hypothesized that imbalance between the procoagulant effects of thrombin and the anticoagulant effects of plasmin may increase the risk that small fibrin clots may be inadequately lysed and may persist and extend.

One may postulate that the thrombo-haemorrhagic balance would shift in favour of thrombosis if any of the following prevailed:

1 increased coagulation system activity
2 increased platelet activity
3 decreased fibrinolytic system activity
4 endothelial damage or abnormality.

At present we have little capability to assess endothelial function or dysfunction or those abnormalities of platelet function which predispose to thrombosis. It is therefore proposed to direct the substance of this chapter towards abnormalities affecting the coagulation and fibrinolytic systems.

Inherited thrombophilia

The abnormalities listed in Table 11.1 are associated with an increased tendency to develop thrombosis. All of these disorders appear to represent autosomal dominant traits although their penetrance is variable.

Apart from Protein S deficiency, thrombophilia due to deficiency of a haemostatic component may be described as type 1—due to a quantitative reduction in synthesis of a normal protein; or type 2—due to a qualitative defect in a protein. In type 1 deficiencies, functional and immunological assay results

Table 11.1 Inherited thrombophilia

Antithrombin III deficiency
Protein C deficiency
Protein S deficiency

are concordantly reduced. In type 2 deficiencies, functional assay results are discordantly reduced when compared with immunological assay results.

Antithrombin III deficiency

Antithrombin III neutralizes thrombin and other serine proteases of the intrinsic coagulation system (FXa, FIXa, FXIa, FXIIa). Its speed of action is enhanced in the presence of heparin and to a lesser extent endothelial cell surface heparin-like proteoglycans. Familial ATIII deficient patients described so far have had ATIII levels of 0.4–0.7 U/ml. (Barrowcliffe & Thomas, 1987). In general ATIII levels of greater than 0.8 U/ml are considered unlikely to predispose to thrombosis.

Type 1 ATIII deficiency (reduced ATIII biological activity, reduced ATIII antigen) may be observed in around 2% of young patients (40–45 years or less) with a history of venous thrombo-embolism (Vikijdal *et al.*, 1985). In the general population a prevalence of heterozygous ATIII deficiency of 1/2000 to 1/5000 (Odegard & Abilgaard, 1978; Rosenberg, 1975) has been reported. To date no homozygous type I ATIII deficient patient is known to have survived beyond a few days.

Families with type II ATIII deficiency (reduced activity, but normal antigen levels) are also described (Lane *et al.*, 1987a,b).

Not all individuals with ATIII deficiency will develop thrombosis, but by the age of 50, around 70% will have suffered at least one episode (Thaler & Lechner, 1981). In some, the episodes of venous thrombosis seem to be spontaneous but in many, additional risk factors, for example pregnancy, surgery, trauma or oestrogens, may be identified.

Protein C deficiency

Protein C (PC) is a vitamin K dependent glycoprotein which has to be converted to activated Protein C before it can perform its anticoagulant function. *In vivo*, thrombin converts PC to its activated form in a reaction enhanced by interaction with endothelial cell thrombomodulin. Once evolved, activated Protein C is a potent inhibitor of FVa and FVIIIa. Both of these reactions require Protein S as a co-factor.

Protein C activity in normal volunteers is reported to be 0.61–1.32 U/ml (Bertina *et al.*, 1984). Protein C leveis of 0.55–0.65 U/ml may be consistent with either heterozygous deficiency or the lower end of the normal distribution. In a study using immunologic assays Miletich *et al.* (1987) suggested that only PC levels of less than 0.55 U/ml are highly predictive of heterozygous deficiency. Laboratories must establish their own normal ranges for the particular assay method they are using but in general it is recommended that family studies are performed in the investigation of individuals with PC activity of 0.65 U/ml or less.

Type 1 PC deficiency (reduction in PC activity and in PC antigen) is reported in around 5–8% of young patients with a history of unexplained venous thrombosis (Gladson *et al.*, 1985; Broekmans *et al.*, 1986). Broekmans *et al.* (1983) estimated that the prevalence of heterozygous PC deficiency is about 1 in 16 000. This estimate was based on studying 319 patients with a history of venous thrombosis. Apart from the clinically dominant form of PC deficiency, a clinically recessive form may exist. In a recently reported study in blood donors in St Louis, USA, the prevalence of heterozygous PC deficiency appeared to be as high as 1/300 (Miletich *et al.*, 1987). The reasons for the enormous difference in prevalence of PC deficiency reported by Broekmans *et al.* (1983) and Miletich *et al.* (1987) are at present not entirely clear.

Type II PC deficiency (PC activity reduced, PC antigen normal) has also been described (Bertina *et al.*, 1984).

Clinically, heterozygous PC deficiency resembles ATIII deficiency—but the overall risk of deep vein thrombosis may be less and the incidence of superficial thrombophlebitis may be greater (Broekmans, 1985). In the initial phases of oral anticoagulant therapy or at times of poor anticoagulant control, patients with PC deficiency have an increased tendency to develop coumarin-induced skin necrosis characterized by progressive thrombosis of the microvessels of the skin (McGehee *et al.*, 1984).

Homozygous PC deficiency has been described presenting in the neonate with extensive thrombosis of visceral veins or with purpura fulminans (Marciniak *et al.*, 1985). If not treated, these infants may develop massive and fatal thrombosis (Seligsohn *et al.*, 1984).

Protein S deficiency

Protein S (PS) is necessary for the full anticoagulant effect of activated PC (Walker, 1984). In plasma, PS is partly free and partly bound to C4b-binding protein. About 50% of C4b-binding protein in normal plasma is complexed with about 50% of the PS (Dahlback, 1983). The level of C4b-binding protein determines the relative amounts of bound and free PS. Only free PS functions as a co-factor for activated PC in the inactivation of FVa and FVIIIa. The equilibrium distribution of PS between free and bound forms may regulate the activity of PS.

Deficiency of PS is associated with an increased thrombotic risk. The range of total PS antigen in normal volunteers is reported to be 0.67–1.25 U/ml and free PS antigen 0.23–0.49 U/ml—calculated from concentrations of total PS and total C4b-binding protein (Bertina *et al.*, 1985). Many laboratories prefer to express free PS antigen levels as a percentage of 'normal' free PS levels. This practice is acceptable but great care must be taken to avoid confusion in the expression of PS results. Each laboratory must establish its own normal ranges for total and free PS antigen.

Heterozygous PS deficiency (reduced PS antigen) is clinically similar to PC deficiency. Although first reports suggested that patients with PS deficiency seem not to be at risk of haemorrhagic skin necrosis (Mannucci & Tripodi, 1988) more recently necrosis of the skin induced by coumarin has been described in a patient deficient in PS (Grimaudo *et al.*, 1989). Among young patients with a history of venous thrombosis, PS deficiency seems to be as prevalent as PC deficiency (5–8%) (Gladson *et al.*, 1985; Broekmans *et al.*, 1986).

Recently purpura fulminans has been described in a neonate with homozygous PS deficiency (Mahasandana *et al.*, 1990).

Other possible thrombophilic disorders

A variety of other factors which may be associated with an increased incidence of venous thrombosis have been described (Table 11.2).

Plasminogen deficiency

Patients with hypoplasminogenaemia (type 1 deficiency) or dysplasminogenaemia (type II deficiency) and a history of recurrent venous thrombosis have been described (Dolan *et al.*, 1988; Mannucci *et al.*, 1986; Lottenberg *et al.*, 1985; Aoki *et al.*, 1978; Wohl *et al.*, 1979, 1982). These defects appear to be transmitted as autosomal dominants but in affected families a low percentage of the heterozygotes are symptomatic (Aoki *et al.*, 1978).

Defects in plasminogen activator synthesis or release

Tissue type plasminogen activator (t-PA) is synthesized mainly in vascular endothelium and released into plasma (Bachmann & Kruithof, 1984). Resting

Table 11.2 Disorders which may be associated with increased risk of thrombosis

Plasminogen deficiency
Defects in plasminogen activator synthesis or release
Increased levels of fibrinolytic inhibitors
Dysfibrinogenaemia
Heparin cofactor II deficiency
Increased levels of histidine rich glycoprotein
Factor XII deficiency
Inborn errors of metabolism (e.g. homocystinuria)

levels of t-PA are low but release of t-PA can be stimulated by exercise, DDAVP or venous occlusion.

Approximately 35% of patients with recurrent or idiopathic venous thrombosis have an impaired fibrinolytic response to venous occlusion (Wiman *et al.*, 1985; Juhan-Vague *et al.*, 1987) but in only a minority is this poor fibrinolytic response due to impaired t-PA release.

Increased levels of fibrinolytic inhibitors

Most patients found to have poor fibrinolytic activity following venous occlusion are found on further examination to have elevated levels of plasminogen activator inhibitors (Wiman *et al.*, 1985; Juhan-Vague *et al.*, 1987). Plasminogen activator inhibitor-1 (PAI-1) is synthesized and released by endothelial cells. Elevated levels of PAI-1 are found in a wide variety of clinical conditions. It has proven difficult to assess the relevance of elevated PAI activity in the aetiology of venous thrombo-embolism.

Dysfibrinogenaemia

Worldwide more than 100 families with abnormal fibrinogens are reported (Gralnick, 1983). Only a minority (approximately 10%) of these abnormal fibrinogens are associated with an increased thrombotic risk. Thrombosis in these families may be either venous or arterial.

Heparin cofactor II deficiency; increased levels of histidine rich glycoprotein; Factor XII deficiency

Patients have been reported in whom thrombosis, venous or arterial, has been associated with one of the above inheritable disorders. However, the role of these haemostatic disorders in inherited thrombophilia remains unproven. (Bertina *et al.*, 1987; Engesser *et al.*, 1986).

Inborn errors of metabolism

Patients with inborn errors of metabolism, for example those causing homocysteinaemia, may be at increased risk of thrombosis.

Acquired thrombophilia

The vast majority of thrombotic disorders are not associated with inherited haemostatic risk factors. Although most thrombotic episodes remain unexplained many occur in association with acquired systemic disorders.

Disorders associated with increased blood viscosity, increased platelet activation or endothelial damage may be expected to have an increased incidence of thromboses, but other mechanisms may also be important, for example loss of ATIII in nephrotic syndrome or reduced synthesis of anticoagulant proteins in liver failure.

Increasingly, the most commonly recognized acquired thrombophilic disorder is the presence of the so-called lupus anticoagulant.

Lupus anticoagulant

Lupus anticoagulant and anticardiolipin antibodies are closely related antiphospholipid antibodies which are associated with a range of clinical manifestations (Table 11.3) including recurrent thrombo-embolism (both venous and arterial), recurrent fetal loss and immune thrombocytopenia (ITP) (Lechner, 1987).

These antibodies are frequently associated with false positive syphilis tests and may be associated with the development of other autoantibodies, notably antinuclear antibodies (Harris *et al.*, 1983). About 10% of patients with systemic lupus erythematosus (SLE) can be shown to have lupus anticoagulants but lupus anticoagulants and/or anticardiolipin antibodies may be found in association with other disorders (Table 11.4), following drug exposure and sometimes in patients with no detectable underlying disease (Primary antiphospholipid syndrome, Harris, 1987).

The mechanisms of thrombosis in patients with lupus anticoagulants remain unclear; furthermore it is uncertain whether lupus anticoagulants and/or anticardiolipin antibodies developing in patients following drug exposure or viral infection are associated with an increased risk of thrombosis.

Table 11.3 Clinical associations of lupus anticoagulant and anticardiolipin antibodies

Venous thrombosis
DVT/PTE
Renal, hepatic, retinal veins
Pulmonary hypertension
Arterial thrombosis
Leg arteries/axillary arteries
Cerebral/visceral/retinal arteries
Coronary arteries
Recurrent fetal loss
Thrombocytopenia
Dermatological manifestations
Livedo reticularis

Table 11.4 Occurrence of lupus anticoagulants and anticardiolipin antibodies

Systemic lupus erythematosus
Other autoimmune disorders
Lymphoproliferative disorders
Viral infection
Following drug exposure (e.g. hydralazine, chlorpromazine)
Primary antiphospholipid syndrome

Investigation of patients with thrombosis

It is generally agreed that the most important candidates for detailed haemostatic investigation and thrombophilia screening are patients who develop 'unexplained' thrombo-embolism under the age of 40–45 years or arterial thrombosis under the age of 30. If investigation is limited strictly to this group, however, the diagnosis will be missed in those patients who develop their first thrombosis at a later age.

It is suggested that the desirability of thrombophilia screening must be assessed on an individual patient basis but that patients who present in any of the categories listed in Table 11.5 should be given special consideration.

Initial investigations

Investigation must commence with a full medical history, a past history, and a drug history. A negative family history does not exclude an inherited abnormality—the defects have low penetrance and fresh mutations occur. The initial investigations, however, must start with the exclusion of common acquired causes of thrombosis, for example malignancy, myeloproliferative disease, hyperlipidaemia, diabetes mellitus and chronic liver disease.

Patients showing an abnormality in any of the initial tests require more detailed investigation of the specific abnormality but it is not the purpose of this chapter to describe these investigations.

Table 11.5 Patients to investigate for thrombophilia

Venous thrombo-embolism before the age of 40–45 years
Recurrent venous thrombosis or thrombophlebitis
Thrombosis in an unusual site, e.g. mesenteric vein, cerebral vein, etc.
Unexplained neonatal thrombosis
Skin necrosis, particularly if on coumarins
Arterial thrombosis before the age of 30
Relatives of patients with thrombophilic abnormality
Patients with clear family history of venous thrombosis
Unexplained prolonged activated partial thromboplastin time
Patients with recurrent fetal loss, ITP or SLE

Screening for inherited thrombophilia

The screening tests are aimed at detecting the most frequent and well-established causes of thrombophilia, i.e. deficiencies or dysfunctions of antithrombin III (ATIII), Protein C (PC) or Protein S (PS). These 'screening' tests should include functional assays capable of detecting both type I and type II abnormalities. To date, however, this goal has not been achieved for protein S as there are at present no widely available well-standardized functional assays for protein S. Tests to detect the presence of lupus anticoagulants must also be included at an early stage of investigation. Tests for plasminogen (Plg) deficiency and fibrinogen deficiency or dysfunction are also usually performed in this first level of investigation.

Table 11.6 lists those tests which should be readily available in all Health Areas to screen for the commoner causes of thrombophilia. Some laboratories may wish to extend their service to include immunological tests to allow them to discriminate between type I and type II defects. However, since immunological assays will not detect type II defects, laboratories should not depend on this type of assay alone.

Screening tests for lupus anticoagulants

Although the presence of a lupus anticoagulant may be suspected in patients with unexplained prolongation of the APTT, the APTT alone is insufficient to detect all of these antibodies and other tests such as the kaolin clotting time, the dilute Russell's Viper Venom time and platelet correction procedures should be employed. In addition the presence of anticardiolipin antibodies (IgG and IgM) should be sought.

The methodological problems of detecting lupus anticoagulant will be discussed in a future *Guidelines* document.

Tests for other possible thrombophilic disorders

If no abnormalities are detected in the initial screening tests, consideration may

Table 11.6 Thrombophilia screening tests

Full blood count, film, platelet count
Prothrombin time
Activated partial thromboplastin time
Thrombin time
Reptilase time
Antithrombin III—functional, chromogenic assay
Protein C—functional, chromogenic or clotting assay
Plasminogen—functional, chromogenic assay
Protein S—total and free protein S, ELISA
Lupus anticoagulant screening tests

be given to referring the patient to a centre with a special interest in the investigation of thrombosis. These centres offer a range of additional tests including those listed in Table 11.7.

When should patients be studied?

As far as possible, detailed investigation of thrombophilia is best avoided in the acute post-thrombotic stage. One must also bear in mind that heparin therapy reduces plasma levels of functional ATIII and that because PC and PS are vitamin K dependent their levels are lowered by oral anticoagulants. If laboratories wish to diagnose Protein C and Protein S deficiency in individuals receiving oral anticoagulants, it is necessary to compare values with other vitamin K dependent clotting factors measured on the same plasma sample. An important prerequisite therefore is the establishment of a 'normal range' of vitamin K dependent factors during stable anticoagulant therapy. This may be outside the scope of smaller laboratories.

Levels of the inhibitors of coagulation may change during normal pregnancy. Protein C antigen levels may be slightly elevated (Mannucci *et al.*, 1984) or remain unaltered. After delivery PC antigen levels are elevated (Mannucci *et al.*, 1984). In contrast, PS levels are significantly reduced during pregnancy and in the puerperium (Comp *et al.*, 1986). Antithrombin III levels are in the normal range in normal pregnancy (Weenink *et al.*, 1982). Oral contraceptives cause a reduction in total and free PS levels (Boerger *et al.*, 1987) a reduction in ATIII levels but no change in PC activity (Cohen *et al.*, 1988). Wherever possible results should be confirmed when the patient is neither pregnant nor taking oral contraceptives.

Family studies

Investigations should be extended to include key family members of patients found to have defects. If possible, parents, siblings and children of the propositus should be encouraged to attend for testing.

Table 11.7 Additional tests for thrombophilia

Fibrinolytic tests before and after stimulation, i.e. venous occlusion (10 minutes or 15 minutes) or DDAVP
fibrin plate
euglobulin lysis time
t-PA—functional assay, chromogenic
PAI—functional assay, chromogenic
Heparin cofactor II—functional assay

Management of individuals with thrombophilia

Acute thrombotic episodes

Thrombotic episodes occurring in patients with thrombophilia should be treated as in patients without documented haemostatic risk factors. Thrombolytic therapy may be considered but usually initial treatment will be with heparin. Patients with ATIII deficiency may be difficult to heparinize and require higher doses of heparin. ATIII levels may further decrease on heparin.

In ATIII deficient patients replacement therapy with ATIII concentrate may be beneficial. At present concentrates of Protein C or Protein S are not widely available for clinical use.

Vitamin K antagonists should be introduced carefully with no loading dose and overlapped with heparin therapy for around 7–10 days.

Prophylaxis against thrombosis

Patients with thrombophilic defects should be given general advice about minimizing their risk of thrombosis—i.e. dietary advice, avoidance of long periods of immobility, etc. Women should, if possible, avoid oestrogen-containing oral contraceptives and hormone replacement therapy. All patients should be warned that they may require special treatment in situations of increased thrombotic risk such as trauma, surgery or pregnancy.

PREVENTION OF FURTHER THROMBOSIS

Careful consideration must be given to the future management of patients with thrombophilia who have already suffered an episode of thrombosis or thrombophlebitis. The risks and the benefits of long-term anticoagulants must be assessed on an individual patient basis taking into account the nature and degree of the thrombophilic defect, other thrombotic 'risk factors' which the patient may have and the circumstances of past thrombotic events. In general ATIII deficiency seems to constitute a greater risk of major thrombosis than, for example, PC or PS deficiency. Patients who have had an apparently spontaneous thrombotic event (not associated with pregnancy, oral contraceptives or surgery) may be viewed to be more likely to have a further spontaneous event than those in whom an obvious 'trigger' was identified.

It is impossible to give 'blanket' advice about the management of these patients: some (those with ATIII deficiency and a history of spontaneous thrombosis) should usually be offered long-term anticoagulation, whilst others (for example women with PC deficiency and a single pregnancy-associated thrombosis) do not usually require long-term anticoagulation if they have no other thrombotic risk factors. Women of childbearing age who are offered long-term anticoagulation must, from the outset, be counselled about the risks of anticoagulant drugs in pregnancy.

Anabolic steroids, such as stanozolol and danazol, stimulate the synthesis of endogenous ATIII and PC and have been used with some success in patients with heterozygous deficiencies. However these agents may have undesirable side effects, particularly in women, if used long-term and they should not at present be considered as an alternative to anticoagulation in the majority of patients.

It must be emphasized that each patient has to be considered on an individual basis. Clinicians dealing with these patients may in some circumstances wish to discuss the management of individual patients with centres with a specialist interest in thrombophilia. Patients not on long-term anticoagulants must be offered short-term prophylaxis to cover situations of increased thrombotic risk.

SPECIAL THROMBOTIC RISK SITUATIONS

Patients with thrombophilia, and their families, must be aware of the requirement for additional therapy in situations where the risk of thrombosis is increased, for example trauma, prolonged immobilization, surgery and pregnancy. In these situations patients should be offered short-term anticoagulation or replacement therapy if they are not already on long-term therapy.

ASYMPTOMATIC FAMILY MEMBERS

In families with inherited thrombophilia, only a proportion of heterozygotes develop thrombosis. It is, therefore, unjustifiable to put family members on prophylactic anticoagulants solely on the basis of having a defect. It is, however, essential that these asymptomatic family members are carefully counselled with respect to their defect and offered short-term prophylaxis in special situations of extra thrombotic risk.

Pregnancy

Pregnancy presents special problems for women with ATIII, PC or PS deficiency or with a lupus anticoagulant. The incidence of deep vein thrombosis associated with pregnancy is high in women with inherited thrombophilia if no prophylaxis is given. Wherever possible affected women should be counselled about their problems before pregnancy and should understand the limitations and risks of any therapy which may be offered.

Warfarin may be teratogenic during the first trimester, resulting in warfarin embryopathy and it is associated with an increased risk of fetal haemorrhage as pregnancy progresses. Women must be warned about the dangers of becoming pregnant while on oral anticoagulants. Where anticoagulation is deemed essential intravenous or self-administered subcutaneous heparin, in adjusted doses, should be considered. However, long-term heparin administration carries a risk of maternal osteoporosis and some clinicians choose to use warfarin during the second and early third trimesters. Oral anticoagulants should if possible be avoided during the first trimester and if used during the mid part of the pregnancy be replaced by heparin at around 36 weeks.

Women who have one of these deficiencies (ATIII, PC or PS) and who have already had a thrombosis require anticoagulation during pregnancy. Women with ATIII deficiency require full anticoagulation from conception onwards. Women with Protein C deficiency, if their previous event was in late pregnancy or the puerperium and if they have had no 'spontaneous' events, probably require less aggressive anticoagulation and it is suggested that in them prophylactic doses of heparin 5000 IU subcutaneously 12 hourly may suffice during the first and perhaps the second trimester. Thereafter full therapeutic doses of heparin should be introduced. The management of PS deficiency is less clear but in general should usually be similar to that of PC deficiency.

The incidence of thrombosis in families known to have ATIII, PC or PS deficiency is very variable and women who have had no previous thrombosis but who are known to have a defect require individual consideration. Since the risk of thrombosis associated with pregnancy in ATIII deficient women seems to be very high, these women require anticoagulation from conception onwards. It is more difficult at present to advise about the management of asymptomatic PC or PS deficient women in pregnancy as no ideal regimen exists. Each woman must be considered on an individual basis.

Replacement of deficient inhibitors with concentrates (where available) is useful at the time of delivery. In patients with ATIII deficiency, ATIII concentrate should be used to cover delivery. Plasma levels of ATIII should, if possible, be maintained betwen 80% and 120% on the day of delivery to allow heparin to be reduced to prophylactic doses only at this time of maximum haemostatic challenge. In these women, 0.75–0.80 units/kg infused ATIII may be expected to raise their plasma ATIII level by 1%. In patients with any of the above deficiencies, anticoagulation should be continued for at least 3 months post partum. Warfarin may be introduced (under heparin cover) 48–72 hours after delivery.

A sample of blood should be obtained from the baby's father (prior to the delivery) for thrombophilic testing so that possible homozygotes or multiple defects may be anticipated. At birth a blood sample should be sent from the baby for thrombophilia screening tests. Occasionally replacement therapy with concentrates or plasma may be necessary in the neonate if he/she develops evidence of thrombosis or is 'sick' or severely preterm.

Women with plasminogen deficiency have not been reported to have an increased incidence of thrombosis in pregnancy perhaps because plasminogen levels increase during pregnancy.

The management of pregnancy in women with lupus anticoagulants is difficult and is currently the subject of study. At present it is suggested that these women may be best managed in centres with previous experience of managing these problematic patients.

It must be stressed that these are general guidelines only; each patient must be considered on on individual basis. Information about the management of women with thrombophilia is continuously being collected. In most instances it is advised that the management of pregnancy in women with these defects should be discussed with centres who have previous experience and expertise.

References

Aoki N., Moroi M., Sakata Y., Yoshida N. & Matsuda M. (1978) Abnormal plasminogen. A hereditary abnormality found in a patient with recurrent thrombosis. *Journal of Clinical Investigation* **61**, 1186–1195.

Bachmann F. & Kruithof E.K.O. (1984) Tissue plasminogen activator: chemical and physiological aspects. *Seminars in Thrombosis and Haemostasis* **10**, 6–17.

Barrowcliffe T.W., Thomas D.P. (1987) Antithrombin III and heparin. In Bloom A.L. & Thomas D.P. (eds) *Haemostasis and Thrombosis*, pp. 849–869 Churchill Livingstone, Edinburgh.

Bauer K.A. & Rosenberg R.D. (1987) The pathophysiology of the prethrombotic state in humans: Insights gained from studies using markers of haemostatic system activation. *Blood* **70**, 343–350.

Bertina R.M., Broekmans A.W., Krommenhoek-van Es. C. & van Wijngaarden A. (1984) The use of a functional and immunological assay for plasma Protein C in the study of the heterogeneity of congenital Protein C deficiency. *Thrombosis and Haemostasis* **51**, 1–5.

Bertina R.M., Reinalda-Poot J.H., van Wijngaarden A., Poort S.R. & Bom V.J. (1985) Determination of plasma Protein S, the protein co-factor of activated Protein C. *Thrombosis and Haemostasis* **53**, 268–272.

Bertina R.M., van der Linden I.K., Engesser L., Muller H.P. & Brommer E.J.P. (1987) Hereditary heparin cofactor II deficiency and the risk of development of thrombosis. *Thrombosis and Haemostasis* **57**, 196–200.

Boerger L.M., Morris P.C., Thurnae G.R., Esmon C.T. & Comp P.C. (1987) Oral contraceptives and gender affect Protein S status. *Blood* **69**, 692–694.

Broekmans A.W. (1985) Hereditary Protein C deficiency. *Haemostasis* **15**, 233–240.

Broekmans A.W., van der Linden I.K., Veltkamp J.J. & Bertina R.M. (1983) Prevalence of isolated Protein C deficiency in patients with venous thrombotic disease and in the population. *Thrombosis and Haemostasis* **50**, 350.

Broekmans A.W., van der Linden I.K., Jansen-Koster Y. & Bertina R.M. (1986) Prevalence of Protein C (PC) and Protein S (PS) deficiency in patients with thrombotic disease. *Thrombosis Research suppl VI*, 135.

Cohen H., Mackie I.J., Walshe K., Gillmer M.D.G. & Machin S.J. (1988) A comparison of the effects of two triphasic oral contraceptives on haemostasis. *British Journal of Haematology* **69**, 259–263.

Comp P.C., Thurnau G.R., Welsh J. & Esmon C.T. (1986) Functional and immunologic Protein S levels are decreased during pregnancy. *Blood* **68**, 881–885.

Dahlback B. (1983) Purification of human C4b-binding Protein and formation of its complex with vitamin K dependent Protein S. *Biochemical Journal* **209**, 847–856.

Dolan G., Greaves M., Cooper P. & Preston F.E. (1988) Thrombovascular disease and familial plasminogen deficiency: A report of three kindreds. *British Journal of Haematology* **70**, 417–421.

Engesser L., Brommer E.J.P. & Briet E. (1986) Elevated levels of histidine-rich glycoProtein in patients with thrombophilia. *Fibrinolysis (Abstracts of the 8th International Congress on Fibrinolysis)* Abstract No. 161.

Gladson C.L., Griffin J.H., Hach V., Beck K.H. & Scharrer I. (1985) The incidence of Protein C and Protein S deficiency in young thrombotic patients. *Blood* **66**, (suppl 1) 350.

Gralnick H.R. (1983) Congenital disorders of fibrinogen. Williams W.J., Beutler E., Ersley A.J. & Lichtman M.A. (eds) *Haematology*. pp. 1399–1410 McGraw-Hill, New York.

Grimaudo V., Gueissaz F., Hauert J., Sarraj A., Kruithof E.K.O. & Bachmann F. (1989) Necrosis of skin induced by coumarin in a patient deficient in Protein S. *British Medical Journal* **298**, 233–234.

Harris E.N. (1987) Syndrome of the Black Swan. *British Journal of Rheumatology* **1**, 324.

Harris E.N., Gharavi A.E., Boey M.L., Patel B.M., Mackworth-Young C.G., Loizou S. & Hughes G.R.V. (1983) Anticardiolipin antibodies: detection by radioimmunoassay and association with thrombosis in systemic lupus erythematosus. *Lancet* **ii**, 1211–1214.

Juhan-Vague I., Valdier J., Alessi M.C. *et al.* (1987) Deficient t-PA release and elevated PA inhibitor levels in patients with spontaneous or recurrent deep venous thrombosis. *Thrombosis and Haemostasis* **57**, 67–72.

Lane D.A., Flynn A. Ireland H., Erdjument H., Samson D. & Thompson E. (1987a) Antithrombin III Northwick Park: demonstration of an inactive high MW complex with increased affinity for heparin. *British Journal of Haematology* **65**, 451–456.

Lane D.A., Lowe G.D.O., Flynn A., Thompson E., Ireland H. & Erdjument H. (1987b) Antithrombin III Glasgow: A variant with increased heparin affinity and reduced ability to inactivate thrombin, associated with familial thrombosis. *British Journal of Haematology* **66**, 523–527.

Lechner K., (1987) Lupus anticoagulants and thrombosis. In Verstraete M., Vermylen J., Lijnen R. & Arnout J. (eds) *Thrombosis and Haemostasis* pp. 525–547 Leuven University Press.

Lottenberg R., Dolly F.R. & Kitchens C.S. (1985) Recurrent thromboembolic disease and pulmonary hypertension associated with severe hypoplasminogenaemia. *American Journal of Haematology* **19**, 181–195.

McGehee W.G., Klotz T.A., Epstein D.J. & Rapaport S.I. (1984) Coumarin necrosis associated with hereditary Protein C deficiency. *Annals of Internal Medicine* **101**, 59–60.

Mahasandana C., Suvatte V., Marlar R.A., Manco-Johnson M.J., Jacobson L.J. & Hathaway W.E. (1990) Neonatal purupura fulminans associated with homozygous Protein S deficiency. *Lancet* **335**, 61–62.

Mannucci P.M., Vigano S., Bottasso B., Candotti G., Borretti B., Rossi E. & Pardi G. (1984) Protein C Ag during pregnancy, delivery and puerperium. *Thrombosis and Haemostasis* **52**, 217.

Mannucci P.M., Kluft C., Traas D.W., Seveso P. & D'Angelo A. (1986) Congenital plasminogen deficiency associated with venous thromboembolism: therapeutic trial with stanozolol. *British Journal of Haematology* **63**, 753–759.

Mannucci P.M. & Tripodi A. (1988) Inherited factors in thrombosis. *Blood Reviews*. **2**, 27–35.

Marciniak E., Wilson H.D. & Marlar R.A. (1985) Neonatal purpura fulminans: a genetic disorder related to the absence of Protein C in blood. *Blood* **65**, 15–20.

Miletich J., Sherman L. & Broze G. (1987) Absence of thrombosis in subjects with heterozygous Protein C deficiency. *New England Journal of Medicine* **317**, 991–995.

Odegard O.R. & Abilgaard U. (1978) Antithrombin III: critical review of assay methods. Significance of variations in health and disease. *Haemostasis* **7**, 127–134.

Rosenberg R.D. (1975) Action and interaction of antithrombin and heparin. *New England Journal of Medicine* **16**, 146–151.

Seligsohn U., Berger A., Abend M., Rubin L., Attias D., Zivelin A. & Rapaport S.I. (1984) Homozygous Protein C deficiency manifested by massive thrombosis in the newborn. *New England Journal of Medicine* **310**, 559–582.

Thaler E. & Lechner K. (1981) Antithrombin III deficiency and thromboembolism. *Clinics in Haematology* **10**, 369–390.

Vikijdal R., Korninger C., Kyrle P.A., Niessner M., Pabinger I., Thaler E. & Lechner K. (1985) The prevalence of hereditary antithrombin III deficiency in patients with a history of venous thromboembolism. *Thrombosis and Haemostasis* **54**, 744–745.

Walker F.J. (1984) Protein S and the regulation of activated Protein C. *Seminars in Thrombosis and Haemostasis* **10**, 131–138.

Weenink G.H., Treffers P.E., Kahle L.H. & Ten Cate J.W. (1982) Antithrombin III in normal pregnancy. *Thrombosis Research* **26**, 281–287.

Wiman B., Ljunberg B., Chimielewska J., Urden G., Blomback M. & Johnsson H. (1985) The role of the fibrinolytic system in deep vein thrombosis. *Journal of Laboratory and Clinical Medicine* **105**, 265–270.

Wohl R.C., Summaria L. & Robbins K.C. (1979) Physiological activation of the human fibrinolytic system. Isolation and characterization of human plasminogen variants. Chicago I and Chicago II. *Journal of Biological Chemistry* **254**, 9063–9069.

Wohl R.C., Summaria L. & Robbins K.C. (1982) Human plasminogen variant. Chicago III. *Thrombosis and Haemostasis* **48**, 146–152.

12 Hospital Blood Bank Documentation and Procedures

Prepared by the
Blood Transfusion Task Force

The purpose of this chapter is to define minimum requirements for documentation in relation to blood transfusion. No attempt is made to prescribe the format in which the information is stored as experience has shown a very wide variety of record keeping systems in use in this country. The principles on which the Task Force has based its recommendations are as follows.

1 The patient identification must be unique.

2 There must be a clear link between each stage in the procedure from the collection of the sample to the connection of the unit for transfusion.

3 That it be possible to trace every stage, the time at which it occurred and the individuals who were involved. Standard operating procedures must be followed in both clinical and laboratory areas.

The Task Force strongly recommends the establishment of a local joint working party to talk through and agree procedures so that the procedures are agreed by all staff involved in direct patient care.

The generation of the request

A request to the blood transfusion laboratory for grouping and/or compatibility testing should be made on a form which contains the following information:

The patient's full surname, correctly spelt
Forename(s) (initials are not sufficient)
The date of birth (a year of birth or age is not sufficient)
The hospital number
Sex

All these pieces of information are essential and consideration should be given to refusing to accept specimens and/or request forms which do not have the information required to identify the individual uniquely.

In situations where a unique number is not available the use of the patient's address may be of benefit and space should be made available for its inclusion.

Alternatively where the patient cannot be identified an Accident and Emergency Department unique number may be used.

It is desirable that the request form should give the destination of the report and that it should contain information about the previous transfusion and obstetric history of the patient. This is usually requested in a series of questions to which simple answers may be entered. Responsibility for completion of the transfusion request form must be accepted by the medical officer. The request form, together with a sample of blood labelled with *the same complete patient identification as on the request form*, is sent to the laboratory.

A special problem of identification may exist in relation to samples from mother and newborn baby received separately. Attention is drawn to this problem but it is felt that local requirements vary so much that guidelines cannot be given other than that an agreed policy for identifying specimens from mother and baby must be documented.

Because transcription is the most common source of error in relation to blood transfusion it is common practice in a number of blood transfusion laboratories to make use of three or four-part NCR stationery so that the top copy of the transfusion request becomes the blood group report and the subsequent copies are used for identifying compatible blood and for serving as the laboratory master record. This may not be necessary in departments where reports are computer generated. For example see Figure 12.1.

The layout of the information on the form may vary but it is recommended that the patient identification and the destination of the report should be contained within a box and that the patient information should appear in a regular pattern which is repeated throughout the patient's record.

Collection of the patient sample

Many hospitals insist that the request form is not only signed by a member of the medical staff but the specimen is also collected by the same member of the medical staff.

In the view of the Task Force, a properly constituted team of phlebotomists who have been properly trained, who have signed an undertaking which makes their responsibilities absolutely clear and who are responsible to a member of the consultant staff of the hospital, may be trusted with the collection of blood for transfusion. Attention is drawn to the guide lines on phlebotomists drawn up by the Royal College of Pathologists*. It is emphasized that the decision whether or not they should be used must be a local one.

The Task Force makes the following recommendations.

* Paper on training of phlebotomists, 1989. Available from The College Secretary, The Royal College of Pathologists, 2 Carlton House Terrace, London SW1Y 5AF.

(a)

HOSPITAL	BLOOD GROUP (If known)	SURNAME	FORENAME(S)	SEX M/F
WARD	PREVIOUS LAB. No.	UNIT No.	DATE OF BIRTH	
CONSULTANT	PREVIOUS TRANSFUSIONS YES/NO	ADDRESS		
MEDICAL OFFICER (SIG.)	ATYPICAL ANTIBODIES YES/ NONE KNOWN	Affix Addressograph Labels to all copies	Sample must be labelled with Name, Date of Birth, also Unit No. where known	
TIME AND DATE OF REQUEST	DETAILS OF ABOVE	DIAGNOSIS AND REASON FOR REQUEST		

INDICATE REQUIREMENTS	GROUP AND SAVE SERUM	IF BLOOD REQUIRED, STATE	TIME NEEDED	QUANTITY OF UNITS	WHOLE BLOOD
	DIRECT COOMBS		DATE NEEDED		BLOOD AS PACKED CELLS

FOR LABORATORY USE ONLY									WARD USE		
LAB. No.		DATE	UNITS COMPATIBLE	GROUP	EXPIRY DATE	WHOLE BLOOD	PACKED CELLS	TIME GIVEN	DATE GIVEN	SIG.
PROVISIONAL BLOOD GROUP	" " Rh "D"									
CONFIRMED BLOOD GROUP	" " Rh "D"									
ATYPICAL ANTIBODIES										
DIRECT COOMBS										

BLOOD TRANSFUSION REQUEST FORM

(b)

HOSPITAL	BLOOD GROUP (If known)	SURNAME	FORENAME(S)	SEX M/F
WARD	PREVIOUS LAB. No.	UNIT No.	DATE OF BIRTH	
CONSULTANT	PREVIOUS TRANSFUSIONS YES/NO	ADDRESS		
MEDICAL OFFICER (SIG.)	ATYPICAL ANTIBODIES YES/ NONE KNOWN	Affix Addressograph Labels to all copies	Sample must be labelled with Name, Date of Birth, also Unit No. where known	
TIME AND DATE OF REQUEST	DETAILS OF ABOVE	DIAGNOSIS AND REASON FOR REQUEST		

INDICATE REQUIREMENTS	GROUP AND SAVE SERUM	IF BLOOD REQUIRED, STATE	TIME NEEDED	QUANTITY OF UNITS	WHOLE BLOOD
	DIRECT COOMBS		DATE NEEDED		BLOOD AS PACKED CELLS

FOR LABORATORY USE ONLY								X-MATCH RESULTS				
LAB. No.		DATE	UNITS COMPATIBLE	GROUP	EXPIRY DATE	WHOLE BLOOD	PACKED CELLS	RT SAL	37°C SAL	ALB	IDC	PAP
PROVISIONAL BLOOD GROUP	" " Rh "D"											
CONFIRMED BLOOD GROUP	" " Rh "D"											
ATYPICAL ANTIBODIES												
DIRECT COOMBS												
COMMENTS								X-MATCH TIME				SIG.

Fig. 12.1 Blood transfusion request form. (a) Top copy; (b) lower copy.

1 Whenever possible patients should be asked to identify themselves verbally; and they should be given an identification bracelet or indelible skin marking.

2 The collection of the blood, dispersal into containers and labelling of the containers must be carried out individually for each patient, in one continuous uninterrupted operation. Addressograph labels should not be used on sample containers. If local practice dictates that dimensions and anticoagulant content of tubes are critical this should be stated in the purchasing specification.

3 The request form or the sample container or both should be signed by the person collecting the blood.

4 It should be mandatory in the case of unconscious patients that the request be signed and the sample taken by the same medical officer. In the case of unconscious casualties and for major disasters a unique numbering and labelling system must be available in the Accident and Emergency Department.†

Supply of blood from the transfusion centre

Blood products are received from the Transfusion Centre having been selected, grouped and screened. The blood pack label contains the following essential information:

The ABO and Rh (D) group
The date of expiry
A unique number
A product identification

Some or all of this information may be in bar code format for direct computer input.

It is essential that a record is available which shows the details of the products received and the eventual fate of each. This may be kept as a register which is also used as a record of the blood issued.

Each laboratory should record:

the date on which the unit was received,
the ABO and Rh (D) group,
the date of expiry,
the unique number,
the patient(s) to whom it was allocated,
the patient to whom it was given,
the date on which it was given,
details of manipulation prior to transfusion (e.g. laboratory filtration or washing),
a record of its alternative disposal.

This information is essential but need not be kept in one place provided that the history of an individual unit can be traced. See also Chapter 13.

† Wood J.K., Nolan S., Blecher T.E. *et al.* (1990) The M1 Kegworth aircraft disaster—experience in three blood transfusion laboratories. *Clinical and Laboratory Haematology* **12**, 1–7.

Grouping and compatibility testing within the laboratory

It is essential that standard operating procedures are followed.

When the blood sample is received in the blood transfusion laboratory, if the serum is to be separated from the cells this procedure must be treated with great respect. The sample container, when ready for separation, should be placed in a numbered rack and a second container, identically labelled and dated, placed in the rack beside it. Serum is then transferred and the labels matched. These containers should be kept together until the grouping procedure is carried out.

Although it is desirable that grouping should be carried out in batches and compatibility testing should be carried out as a routine exercise, inevitably a percentage of the work is of an emergency nature. It is important that the documentation should allow for these two, often different, procedures. Under ideal circumstances all groupings on patients' blood will be put up in batches with appropriate controls. It is good practice in manual grouping that the cell group and the serum group should be determined by different members of staff and the results collated afterwards. It is necessary that an adequate record of the grouping procedures should be retained and this may conveniently be done by using the worksheet as a permanent document. This will prevent transcription errors.

An alternative approach is to keep a book in which all groups carried out are entered. In either case the worksheet should be retained and should be identified by the date, the time of day, and the name of the person carrying out the work.

If the results are interpreted by someone other than the person performing the test his or her name should also be recorded. Working documents should be retained for 11 years to meet the requirements of the Consumer Protection Act, 1987. There is evidence that diseases with long incubation periods may be transmitted by blood products. It is essential to be able to trace such donors to remove them from the donor panel.

There should be a record of source and batch numbers of reagents used.

Emergency compatibility testing may require that an emergency group is carried out. This may have to be performed by an alternative technique at the time that the crossmatch is carried out, possibly by the same person. Details of this emergency group must be recorded. This may either be done in a book kept for that purpose or alternatively the information may be recorded on the Blood Transfusion request/record form.

Compatibility testing

Information concerning the compatibility testing of blood for a particular patient must be recorded. It may be recorded on a special compatibility testing sheet which contains information about compatibility testing for several patients at the same time. Alternatively or in addition it may be recorded on a blood transfusion compatibility form either as part of an integral blood transfusion request form or as a report issued by the laboratory. Whatever type of documentation is used the following information must be recorded:

the date and time that the procedure was carried out
the person who carried it out
the identification of the patient
the ABO and Rh (D) group of the patient and the donor blood
the unique donation number
the result of the compatibility testing by each technique used

This last item of information need not form part of the compatibility report.

Arrangements should ensure that the compatibility report and the report of the blood group, if separate, become available to the clinical staff in charge of the patient as quickly as possible. This means either a rapid courier service to the ward or alternatively an arrangement whereby these reports are made available when the first unit of blood for that patient is collected.

Collection of compatibility tested blood for transfusion

Blood for transfusion must be stored in specially designated refrigerators, to the specifications as described in the British Standard 4376–1990.* These refrigerators should not be used for any other purpose, should be monitored by use of chart recorders, and should have adequate alarm systems. Wherever possible, separate refrigerators, clearly labelled, should be used for stock blood and compatibility tested blood. Whether in the laboratory, operating theatre or in the clinical area, they must be under the supervision of the consultant in charge of the blood transfusion laboratory, who will arrange regular checks and clearances.

The person collecting the unit should come equipped with documentation which specifies the patient's details. This may be the patient's case record, part of the record containing full identification or a specially designed document (Fig. 12.2).

Blood may be issued on demand by laboratory staff or may be collected directly from the blood refrigerator by designated staff. At the moment of collection the person collecting the blood should satisfy him/herself that identification details relating to the patient and to the unit of blood agree. When blood is issued by the laboratory this will be a two-way exercise between the member of staff issuing the unit and the person collecting it. Where the pack is collected by clinical staff without laboratory intervention the same checking process must apply.

* BS 4376–1990. British Standards Institute, 2 Park Street, London W1A 2BS.

RECEIPT FOR TRANSFUSION FLUIDS

Date ....

Ward/Theatre ....

Please supply the bearer with:

.... unit(s) of whole blood ☐

● Plasma protein fraction batch numbers must be noted here:

Packed red cells ☐

Platelets ☐

● Plasma protein fraction ● ☐

Cryoprecipitate ☐

Factor VIII concentrate ☐

Fibrinogen ☐

Fresh frozen Plasma ☐

Other ☐

(Please specify)

Patient's Details addressograph if available

Surname Forename(s)

Hospital No.

Address

Date of birth

Signed ....

(Must be signed by medical officer, SRN or SEN, not by unqualified staff)

Fig. 12.2 Receipt for transfusion fluids.

There must be a written record retained by the blood transfusion laboratory including (i) identification of the patient for whom blood is collected; (ii) unique donation number of pack collected; (iii) time of collection; (iv) name of person collecting.

The compatibility label

This label should be firmly attached to the unit of blood. It provides information linking the patient's identification to the unit of blood. It should carry the following items:

surname,
forename(s),
date of birth,
hospital number,
patient's group,
unique donor number of pack,
date blood required.

Uncross-matched blood

Circumstances arise when it may be necessary or appropriate to issue blood which has not been compatibility tested. The ABO group of units used in this way must be confirmed before issue and a warning label should be attached to the pack.

Transfusion of different blood group

In situations where this is required a special warning label should be used and the clinical staff contacted by telephone.

Procedures in clinical areas

It is recommended that procedures for the administration of blood products should be agreed between medical and nursing staff and should be implemented as part of a Nursing Code of Practice. The checking procedure for each pack of blood product must be laid down in detail.

The following points are important.

1 The pack should be checked at the patient by two people, one of whom is either a Registered General Nurse or a medical officer. In operating theatres the Operating Department Assistant may take part in the checking procedure with the medical officer. The patient should be asked to identify him/herself unless unconscious or anaesthetized and the information on the following compared:

the patient's identification bracelet or skin marking,
the compatibility report,
the compatibility label on the pack of blood.

2 The ABO and Rh (D) group of the pack should be checked against the blood group report in the case record and the compatibility label on the pack itself.

3 The blood should be examined for any signs of discoloration or haemolysis and the unit should then be tested for leaks by squeezing firmly.

4 It should be checked that the expiry date on the unit of blood has not been exceeded.

REQUESTED FOR: DOB ABO GROUP Rh(D)

REQUIRED FOR:
AVAILABLE FROM: LAB. NO.

BLOOD/BLOOD PRODUCTS TRANSFUSION PRESCRIPTION

Date/ Time Issued	Product	Blood Group	Pack Number	Medical Officer Ordering	Intended Duration of Infusion	Time Started	Given By	Checked By

COMMENTS:

MATCHING PROCEDURE			
ROUTINE	EMERGENCY	PACK GROUP CHECK ONLY	M LSO Signature

The persons administering the blood must confirm that the identification of the patient, the name and date of birth of the patient on the selected blood pack, and the information on this report (including the blood pack number) all agree; and that the pack is not time-expired.
In the event of a transfusion reaction this report should be returned to the BLOOD BANK along with a REACTION REPORT FORM, all blood packs, plus 20 ml of clotted blood and a 5 ml EDTA blood specimen.
The top copy of this form should be filed in the Patient's Case Sheet and the bottom copy returned to the BLOOD BANK as soon as possible after administration of the required units has been completed.

REQUESTED FOR: DOB ABO GROUP Rh(D)

REQUIRED FOR:
AVAILABLE FROM: LAB. NO.

BLOOD/BLOOD PRODUCTS TRANSFUSION PRESCRIPTION

Date/ Time Issued	Product	Blood Group	Pack Number	Medical Officer Ordering	Intended Duration of Infusion	Time Started	Given By	Checked By

PLEASE RETURN THIS COPY TO
THE BLOOD TRANSFUSION SERVICE
AFTER ADMINISTRATION OF BLOOD

COMMENTS:

MATCHING PROCEDURE			
ROUTINE	EMERGENCY	PACK GROUP CHECK ONLY	M LSO Signature

The persons administering the blood must confirm that the identification of the patient, the name and date of birth of the patient on the selected blood pack, and the information on this report (including the blood pack number) all agree; and that the pack is not time-expired.
In the event of a transfusion reaction this report should be returned to the BLOOD BANK along with a REACTION REPORT FORM, all blood packs, plus 20 ml of clotted blood and a 5 ml EDTA blood specimen.
The top copy of this form should be filed in the Patient's Case Sheet and the bottom copy returned to the BLOOD BANK as soon as possible after administration of the required units has been completed.

Fig. 12.3 Intravenous administration form.

As stated above, each unit of blood transfused must be recorded in the patient's notes on a special intravenous administration form (Fig. 12.3) and in the continuation notes. This is important for medical audit.

On this intravenous administration form should be recorded:

the patient identification details,

the day and the time at which the unit was connected,

the signature of the person connecting it,

the signature of the person checking it.

At the end of the transfusion the amount given is recorded on the fluid balance chart and in the continuation notes, and the time at which it was disconnected is recorded. This document must form a permanent part of the patient record. After disconnection, the plastic pack which contained the unit of blood must be retained for at least 48 hours before being discarded. If during this time there is any indication that a transfusion reaction has taken place it is then available to the blood transfusion laboratory for investigation.

Blood transfusion reactions

The recording of blood transfusion reactions is dependent on the level of awareness of the staff looking after the patient but all staff should be encouraged to report incidents which they consider might be related to the infusion of blood products. It is advisable that a set of instructions relating to blood transfusion reactions should be available at ward level. This would define the degrees of severity of these reactions, offer a list of symptoms and signs to be recorded easily and offer advice on the immediate action to be taken by ward staff. Some hospitals utilize a Transfusion Reaction Request for Investigation form (Fig. 12.4).

Blood products

All products of human origin must be accounted for. These include platelets, gamma globulin, human albumin solutions, Factor VIII, Factor IX, cryoprecipitate, fresh frozen plasma, etc.

Some of these—platelets, cryoprecipitate and fresh frozen plasma—have a unique donation number, others have a common batch number.

It is essential that the use of all blood products is fully documented and that all material issued can be traced from receipt to the eventual utilization.

A recording system similar to that described for blood for transfusion is recommended.

The use of these materials should be recorded by patient, date of administration (time where appropriate) and batch number.

TRANSFUSION DEPARTMENT

CASE No.		
SURNAME		
FORENAME(S)		
[ ] Male [ ] Female	Date of Birth	
Patient's Address		
Hospital	Ward	Consultant

INVESTIGATION OF AN APPARENT BLOOD TRANSFUSION REACTION

REQUIREMENTS: NO TESTING CAN BE DONE WITHOUT THE SAMPLES

1) Donor pack causing reaction, complete with giving set.
2) 10 ml of post-transfusion clotted blood.
   Blood cultures on patient.
3) 5 ml of EDTA (sequestrene) blood.
4) First available MSU after the reaction.

TO BE FILLED IN BY MEDICAL OFFICER RESPONSIBLE FOR THE PATIENT

A. THE PATIENT

Brief synopsis of history prior to transfusions:

Previous transfusion
Reason for transfusion
Pre-transfusion Hb
Symptoms of reaction

Pyrexia [ ]	Rigor [ ]	Lumbar Pain [ ]	Rash [ ]
Hypotension [ ]	Tachycardia [ ]	Haemoglobinuria [ ]	
Vomiting [ ]	Jaundice [ ]	Oliguria/Anuria [ ]	

Volume of urine passed since reaction

Female Patients: Pregnancies: Abortions/Miscarriages:

Atypical Antibodies:

All Patients: Previous transfusion reactions:

B. THE BLOOD PACK

GROUP: Rh(D): Unit Number: Expiry Date:

Date and time taken from blood bank

Was blood warmed before infusion?

Time infusion commenced

Number of units of blood already infused through giving set

Was anything injected into the pack or giving set?

Date and time of reaction

Volume of blood infused (approximately)

*Signed*____________________

Fig. 12.4 Transfusion reaction request for investigation form.

13 Hospital Blood Bank Computing

Prepared by the
Blood Transfusion Task Force

Introduction

The procedures involved in the safe grouping, cross-matching and issue of blood and its products include a large clerical component. The increasing and more complex clinical demands on hospital blood banks have reached the stage where the attendant clerical activity is limiting the time available for productive technical work. The specific requirements of the DHSS circular (HC(84)7) for improved record keeping and stock control arrangements, the introduction of Körner workload statistics and the development of clinical budgeting all serve to compound this problem. Automated data processing is an effective way to redress this imbalance.

Special requirements for blood transfusion

Data processing in the hospital blood bank is concerned with patient records and laboratory activities, as in other laboratories; in addition, the system must provide for strict accountability of blood products and include safety prompts for standard procedures, such as blood grouping and cross-matching, to inhibit the issue of incompatible products. The system should have significant real-time access (for example to answer telephone queries with up-to-date patient laboratory records) and be operational 24 hours a day because of the 'out-of-hours' component.

The benefits of such a system would include improvements in operating efficiency with fast and accurate data retrieval, improvements in the quality of work with rationalization of procedures and incorporation of safety controls at critical stages, and potential staff redeployment as a result of improved productivity and less clerical involvement. Furthermore, computerization of blood transfusion records makes available a greater variety of current statistical data than is possible with manual methods because of the enormous labour required. Once a hospital has accurate statistics on its own transfusion service data base, it would be possible to assess the efficiency of blood usage and determine the effects of any change of policy or procedure.

Minimum guidelines

The purpose of this chapter is to define minimum requirements for automated data processing in the hospital blood transfusion laboratory. No attempt is made to recommend a particular system, but these guidelines should assist in selecting a hardware/software package that will meet basic requirements. Laboratories may wish to supplement the basic system to meet special local needs, for example an antenatal package. A system is envisaged which can interact with the hospital Patient Administration System (PAS), other parts of the haematology laboratory and the Regional Transfusion Centre, and which can accommodate the requirements of satellite laboratories. It must be a multi-user system which is expandable without having to re-write the software. It is suggested that a local working party be set up to monitor the operation of the system and introduce changes where appropriate.

The objectives of the system may be defined as:

1 to reduce clerical involvement by laboratory staff at all stages in the preparation and retrieval of laboratory records;

2 to improve legibility and reduce transcription errors in labels, reports and records;

3 to provide additional checking facilities at critical stages in technical procedures for the selection and issue of blood and blood products for transfusion;

4 to record stages in the procedure, the time and the individuals responsible, as recommended in Chapter 12;

5 to record all blood and blood products received and trace the fate of each unit, as required by HC(84)7;

6 to analyse blood and blood product usage and other blood bank data to provide statistical indicators for the audit of blood transfusion practice (see Appendix);

7 to provide statistics for workload analysis and clinical budgeting.

The system should not require major changes in established work patterns, but it should be flexible enough to provide an incentive for rationalization and to permit growth and development of laboratory activity.

Operational requirements

This section lists the desirable functions that should be included in an optimal blood bank data processing system. Probably no single system at present incorporates all of these functions and the choice of system will depend on local requirements and priorities.

Patient records

These should include patient demographic data, previous transfusion history and relevant laboratory data.

PATIENT DEMOGRAPHIC DATA (from PAS where available)

The essential identification criteria for blood transfusion, as set out in Chapter 12, are unique patient number (UPN), surname, forename(s), date of birth and sex. Some additional information, for example ethnic origin, address, may also be accommodated by some systems. Patient location (report/product destination)—i.e. hospital and/or ward—is essential, as is the identity of the requesting consultant.

If the UPN is not available most systems will allocate a temporary number. However, some users may not accept this as adequate documentation and the system should allow input of additional identification data, for example first line of address or house number and postal code.

For newborn babies it is important to have an identification procedure for distinguishing the baby's blood from that of the mother.

PREVIOUS TRANSFUSION HISTORY

ABO and Rh D group (and dates)
Antibodies, genotypes (and dates)
Pregnancy history (parity, antibodies, haemolytic disease of the newborn)
Blood/components transfused (and dates)
Reason for transfusion (coded)
Remarks, e.g., transfusion reaction, requires washed/filtered red cells (coded)
Other blood bank tests (coded)

There should be a facility to 'flag' certain records, for example irregular antibodies or other special transfusion requirements.

The system should:

1 sort and collate data to give a cumulative patient record for each admission;
2 allow immediate recall by UPN/name on a 24 hour, 7 day a week basis during current admission;
3 provide storage for such records, then cull and archive;
4 integrate with other laboratory systems.

The request

REQUEST ENTRY

The order of entry of patient demographic details to the computer system should reflect the order in which the details are given on the request document.

Any data processing system should accept patient demographics transcribed in full from request documents and subsequently generate reports and cross-match labels containing some or all of this data—in effect to perpetuate the recommended practice of always using the exact details given on the request document. Use of the request document itself as the report form is more difficult and would involve the generation of adhesive backed reports to be stuck to the original document. Rigid adherence to the principle of using exact request details will, however, compromise cumulative report/enquiry facilities offered by many systems, as minor variants in patient request details would lead to each event being treated as appertaining to a different patient.

Laboratories may wish to consider methods of interrogating locally held patient indices on the basis of patient number and/or all or part of surname together with details, such as date of birth or sex, and subsequently updating additional patient demographics held on the computer to reflect current information on the request document. Where no previous record exists of course full data must be entered. Ideally, critical patient demographics should be permanently attached to requesting information and current demographics held in a patient index.

Both approaches have drawbacks within a data processing environment and a compromise may be to service a request on the basis of requesting details only. The system, operated by senior staff, would then merge the request with details appertaining to the relevant patient.

NATURE OF REQUEST

Blood component/products are requested from a list of those available to be defined by the user, with date and time required, and reason for transfusion, specifying the surgical operation where relevant.

The concept of maximum surgical blood order (MSBO, see Chapter 16) based on a locally agreed 'tariff' may be incorporated into the programme for cross-matching; entry of a request exceeding the MSBO should require special authorization.

Tests—of blood group, antibody screen, cross-match, etc.—are selected from a list to be defined by the user.

THE BLOOD SAMPLE

It would be desirable to enter the name of the person taking the sample—by implication the person who identified the patient and labelled the blood sample—together with the time and date of taking.

A laboratory (accession) number—preferably bar-coded—should be assigned to each request and affixed to the corresponding blood sample and all samples derived from it.

Laboratory procedure

The entry of a request signals the start of both analytical and data processing.

Requests may be allocated to different work areas within the laboratory in a variety of ways as determined by the user, for example routine and emergency specimens. The system should allow single analysis, as for emergency requests, and batch analysis for routine work. Routine requests may be listed in the order required (time and date); this is especially useful for organizing cross-matching.

Enquiry about requests received/work in progress should be available by patient UPN or laboratory number.

Production of results

The technologist should be able to key results directly into the system, thus eliminating tedious transcription and possible error. Each result/batch of results should include coded entry of method and reagents used and identity of operator responsible, date and time.

There should be a facility to interface with automated blood group and antibody screening systems, including microplate readers.

BLOOD GROUP (ABO/D)

1 Key in serological reactions for computer derivation of blood group; or
2 enter individual blood groups by keyboard or bar code menu card; or
3 interface with automated blood-grouping machine.

Facility for 1 and 2 to be verified by second operator; automatic checking of controls.

ANTIBODY SCREENING

Coded entry of specificity, titre and immunochemical characteristics, for example IgG class, complement fixation, optimal reaction conditions. Also include coded entry of screening cells and method used.

GENOTYPE

Rh; other blood groups.

CROSS-MATCH

There should be a facility for reserving appropriate units from stock (see below) for cross-matching for a particular patient, for example by entering the patient's UPN against each unit. This should include an automatic check of blood group, irregular antibody compatibility and expiry date.

The system should allow a definable reservation period for cross-matched units and produce a return to stock list.

The entry of cross-match results should be accompanied by an audio-visual prompt to verify the identification of the serum sample used for cross-matching; this may include use of bar-coded laboratory (accession) number for cross-checking against patient entry in computer.

The cross-check should include an auto control and an anti-human globulin control for negative indirect antiglobulin tests.

In special circumstances the system should, on instruction, allow issue of apparently incompatible blood.

After verification of results (see below), a compatibility report (blood group and list of compatible units) and compatibility labels for the blood units can then be printed (see below).

After affixing cross-match labels to compatible units, cross-check unit number on label against corresponding number on blood bag, preferably using bar codes.

The system should ultimately record whether or not a compatible unit was transfused and any adverse transfusion reactions.

URGENT CROSS-MATCH

The system should provide for processing single requests in emergency and allow any approved abbreviation of the standard cross-match procedure where necessary.

It should provide for the issue of uncross-matched O Rh-negative or group specific blood, but only on the basis of a group check of the donor blood unit. These units should be clearly labelled 'NOT CROSS-MATCHED'. There should be a facility for retrospective entry of standard cross-match results on these units.

OTHER BLOOD COMPONENTS

The system should record the issue of other blood components and plasma products. Where ABO compatibility is a consideration (e.g. fresh frozen plasma

(FFP), cryoprecipitate, platelet concentrates), the system should permit overriding of blood group identity (with appropriate record keeping) in accordance with agreed local practice.

OTHER TESTS

To be defined by the user, for example direct anti-globulin test, transfusion reaction work-up, etc. There should be a free text entry field for tests not listed.

Verification

Entry of results requires verification of patient registration data against corresponding details on the sample tested. This check is carried out, as specified in Chapter 12, by a designated, responsible person whose identity is accepted by the system.

There should be a facility for: (i) automatic checking of newly entered results against previous data, e.g., blood group; and (ii) supervisory editing and correction. All corrections must be logged and appropriately authorized.

Reports and labels

The system should be able to produce the laboratory's own style of report and label, according to the guidelines given in Chapter 12.

Reports and labels should be readily available, either singly or in batches, as soon as the results have been verified.

Other hard copy, for example day books, activity logs, 'Blood Bank Register' of cross-matched units, etc. should be available from the system, if required.

Blood bank stock control

All blood products entering the laboratory (from one or more Regional Transfusion Centres—RTCs) must be booked into the system, and the subsequent fate of each unit recorded, for example transfused, returned to RTC, or otherwise disposed of (specify), as required by DHSS circular HC(84)7. A modem link to the RTC may facilitate this procedure by providing automatic notification of deliveries and confirmation of receipt. Information entered against each unit to be defined by the user, for example unit number, product code, blood group, expiry date, entry date. Wherever possible bar-coding should be used.

The following information is essential for stock management and product accountability.

1 Current stock display—showing status of each unit, for example free, modified (specify), reserved (cross-matched), issued for transfusion, transfused, presumed transfused, returned to stock, out-dated, discarded (specify), returned to RTC, otherwise disposed of (specify).
2 A print-out of cross-matched units would assist checking before issue in the same way as the current Blood Bank Register.
3 Available stock summary—numerical summary of available blood products including blood group and expiry date where relevant—to assist allocation of resources and re-ordering.
4 Monthly stock statistics—summary of fate of all blood products received during the month to meet requirements of HC(84)7.

Security controls

All recorded data must be traceable to the person(s) who entered the information.

To ensure that only authorized users have access, a password system is necessary to identify bona fide users and allowable functions. The system should be able to generate reports to monitor this.

All recorded data must be available for hard-copy reproduction. Any change of result must be logged by the system and there must be a reliable way of identifying the authenticity of changes or corrections made in the original records.

If VDUs are situated in public areas (including wards), the system must include a time-out facility to prevent sensitive information being available to non-authorized personnel.

Back-up systems

The system should provide for: (i) duplication of data to appropriate media at regular intervals to safeguard primary data; (ii) back-up when the computer is 'down'—either manual or preferably a mini-computer; there should be easy transfer of data to the main system when it is operating again.

Data storage

A culling system is necessary to manage the quantity of data generated. This should allow the user to keep specific data on-line for ongoing patient management and delete or archive other stored data. In general, records should be accessible in relation to their frequency of use.

Certain data must be selected and time limits set for on-line storage; experience with the system will lead to refinements of initial decisions. The following are guidelines for some data, but compromises may be necessary for on-line storage depending on resources available.

1 ABO/D groups—at least 1 year on line; archive as long as possible (incorporate in hospital PAS).

2 Irregular antibodies/genotype—for life of patient on-line.

3 Compatibility tests/transfused units—2 months on-line; archive at least 8 years.

4 Fate of all units—2 months on-line; archive at least 8 years.

5 Transfusion reactions—for life of patient on-line.

6 'Problem' patients (specify)—for life of patient on-line.

The period of storage should conform to the recommendations of notes concerning 'Preservation and destruction of hospital records' HM(61)73 as amended by HC(80)7.

Concluding remarks

Installing a computer will greatly assist the operation of the blood transfusion laboratory, but it remains the responsibility of the consultant in charge to operate the system for the benefit of the patient and to maintain standards of safe practice and quality assurance. It is inevitable that 'grey areas' will remain, where the computer will not provide the answer, and here the consultant must exercise his/her judgement on the basis of the facts available.

It is recommended that the 'Guideline specification for machine readable labels for use in the UK', prepared by a Regional Transfusion Director's working party, should be followed in designing bar-code labels for any system, and the Secretary (Dr M.M. Fisher, Oxford RTC) should be consulted about codes in current use.

The blood bank computer system must be registered under the Data Protection Act (1984), which requires special arrangements for physical, software and operational security.

Appendix: Analysis of blood product usage and other blood bank data*

The following statistical indicators are of value in the audit of blood transfusion practice.

*Based on Simpson M.B. (1982) Audit criteria for transfusion practice. In Wallas C.H. & Muller V.H. (eds) *The Hospital Transfusion Committee*, pp. 21–60. American Association of Blood Banks, Arlington, Virginia.

ESSENTIAL INDICATORS

Individual patient and unit information. Review all units transfused to a patient and the fate of a particular unit (essential to meet requirements of HC(84)7).

Cross-match to transfused ratio (C:T). Analysis by total number (essential), by consultant, ward, clinical specialty, surgical procedure, emergency versus routine requests (optional).

Out-date rate. Monitored for all blood components/products; analysis by blood group where appropriate.

Workload. As required for DHSS statistics; analysis by consultant, technician, time and day of week (optional).

OPTIONAL INDICATORS

Total components transfused. Whole blood, packed red cells, proportion of red cells transfused as whole blood, leucocyte-poor red cells, washed red cells, frozen red cells, 'fresh' blood, platelet concentrates, apheresis platelets, FFP, cryoprecipitate, human albumin; other blood products as defined by the user.

Total patients transfused. Analysis by blood component as listed above.

Units transfused per patient. Analysis by blood product, consultant, diagnosis, surgical operation.

Units returned unused. Number (%) of units signed out and later returned unused; analysis by consultant, ward, specialty.

Uncross-matched units issued. Number (%) of units issued uncross-matched or after abbreviated pre-transfusion testing; analysis by consultant, ward, diagnosis/surgical procedure.

Late cross-match requests for elective procedures. Number (%) of requests received after laboratory deadline; analysis by consultant, ward, diagnosis/surgical procedure, time and day.

Emergency requests. Number (%) analysed by consultant, ward, diagnosis, distribution by time and day of week; C:T ratio.

Adverse transfusion reactions. Number (%) analysed by type of reaction, including post-transfusion hepatitis.

Distribution of requests. Number (%) analysed by time and day of week; consultant, ward, specialty.

References

Blood transfusion: record keeping and stock control arrangements. DHSS HC(84)7.

Guideline specification for machine readable labels for use in the UK. Report of RTD Working Party, May 1984.

Preservation and destruction of hospital records HM(61)73, as amended by HC(80)7: *Retention of personal health records (for possible use in litigation)*.

14 Compatibility Testing in Hospital Blood Banks

Prepared by the
Blood Transfusion Task Force

Introduction

These guidelines have been revised since first being published in 1987 (BCSH, 1987) to take account of the many comments received from BSH/BBTS members and from international experts on working parties of the ICSH/ISBT Expert Panel on Serology.

The aim of this chapter is to present a *minimum* standard for pre-transfusion compatibility testing. The approach is mainly advisory, although details of important principles and techniques are given. In this review of the guidelines the Working Party has addressed the contentious issue of the cross-match. The continuing unacceptable level of antibody detection failures in external proficiency trials dictates a cautious approach towards omission of the antiglobulin phase of the cross-match for patients with a negative antibody screen. For the first time the guidelines advocate periodic assessment of individual staff competence and regular monitoring of cell washing centrifuges as essential prerequisites for abbreviating the cross-match to a rapid spin procedure.

The design of procedures for emergency situations is particularly difficult as, in the overall interests of the patient, sensitivity may have to be compromised. In this situation two pitfalls must be avoided; the issue of ABO incompatible blood because of inadequate and rushed procedures on the one hand; and failure to supply blood before the patient becomes irreversibly shocked on the other. An element of flexibility must therefore be allowed which requires a high level of training and an understanding of the clinical situation.

General considerations

Safe and efficient blood transfusion practice requires the following procedures.

1 Constant attention to the reliability of reagents and techniques.

2 Elimination of clerical errors; procedures to ensure this is achieved are detailed in Chapters 12 and 13.

3 Consideration of patient's history (e.g. transfusions, pregnancy, drugs), which should be stated on the request form.

4 A satisfactory compatibility procedure, which should include:

(a) accurate ABO and Rh D grouping to ensure (i) ABO compatibility; (ii) use of blood of the same Rh D group, wherever possible; this is particularly important for all female patients up to the age of menopause;

(b) antibody screening of the patient's serum to detect the presence of clinically significant antibodies;

(c) cross-matching the patient's serum against donor red cells.

All staff undertaking the work must be appropriately trained and an objective assessment of technical competence should be instituted and maintained.

All methodology must be detailed as standard operating procedures in a laboratory manual which must be readily available (see Chapter 19).

All laboratories should participate in the National External Quality Assurance Scheme for Blood Group Serology.

General laboratory procedures

Documentation

The safety of blood transfusion depends on accurate patient and sample identification at all stages, starting with taking the blood sample from the patient for compatibility testing and ending with the transfusion of compatible blood—see Chapter 12.

In the laboratory clerical errors can be avoided if the worker performing the compatibility test *double checks* the identity of the patient's sample with the request form and with the compatibility label on the donor units before issuing the blood. Whenever possible, all checks should be made by two responsible persons.

Away from the laboratory it must also be remembered that deaths due to ABO incompatibility may occur because staff give blood to the wrong patient having failed to double check the identity of the patient.

Reagents

Constant attention should be paid to the reliability of reagents. The laboratory must test each new batch of reagents and show that they give the expected reactions with appropriate controls before their introduction into routine use. Furthermore, controls must be included with each batch of tests. The lot numbers of all reagents in use must be documented. Laboratories that lack the resources to evaluate reagents should consult their Regional Transfusion Centre.

All reagents should be used according to the manufacturer's instructions, unless appropriately standardized for alternative methods.

For further information see *Guidelines for reagents for blood group serology and HLA typing* (UKBTS/NIBSC, 1990).

Cell suspension for compatibility testing

For tests at normal ionic strength, red cell samples should be washed and resuspended to 2–3% in 8.5–9.0 g/l sodium chloride, preferably buffered to pH 7.0 ± 0.2 with 0.145 mol/L–0.154 mol/L phosphate salts.

For low ionic strength tests, red cell samples should be washed at least twice in saline and once in low ionic strength solution (LISS) before suspending to 1.5–2.0% in LISS. This is necessary to avoid non-specific uptake of complement by test red cells. Red cells suspended in normal ionic strength saline (NISS) or LISS can only be used for 24 hours after their preparation.

Serum : cell ratios

As a minimum, laboratories should seek to use a serum : cell ratio of 40 : 1. Since the volume of a 'drop' varies according to the type of pipette or dropper bottle, a measured or known drop volume should be used to ensure that appropriate serum : cell ratios are maintained.

NISS and LISS tests

For NISS tests, the serum : cell ratio should be at least 2 vols of serum : 1 vol 2–3% red cells in saline. The minimum incubation time is 45 minutes at 37°C.

For LISS tests, the serum : cell ratio should be 2 vols of serum : 2 vols 1.5–2.0% red cells in LISS. The minimum incubation time is 15 minutes at 37°C.

For direct agglutination tests using NISS or LISS, the incubation phase may be omitted or markedly reduced, provided appropriate centrifugation is used.

Laboratories that use LISS for routine work are well placed to meet urgent compatibility requests. However, where laboratories use NISS tests routinely, it is not recommended that they change to LISS tests for emergency techniques.

Blood samples

Immediately on receipt, laboratory staff must confirm that the blood sample is appropriately labelled and that the information on the sample and request form are identical.

Great care must be taken to identify and label correctly any serum separated from the patient's original blood sample; the serum should be stored at or below −20°C.

If the patient has been transfused with blood products containing red cells since the date of collection of the serum sample in storage, and if that transfusion was given more than 3 days ago, a new blood sample is required for antibody screening and cross-matching to detect the emergence of any new antibodies.

Microplate technology

Laboratories changing from tube to microplate techniques should refer to BCSH guidelines for microplate techniques for liquid phase blood grouping and antibody screening (Chapter 15).

Pretransfusion testing

The ABO and Rh D group must be determined for each specimen received and an antibody screening test performed. Cross-matching of patient's serum and donor red cells should be performed before transfusion.

The observed test results should be compared with those recorded for previous samples. Any discrepancies should be resolved before the issue of blood.

ABO and Rh D grouping

These must be performed by an approved technique with appropriate controls (Appendix 1). If auto or reagent (diluent) controls are positive, great care must be taken in the interpretation of the grouping results, and if necessary advice should be sought from a regional transfusion centre.

ABO grouping. ABO compatibility is an essential requirement of safe transfusion practice. Correct interpretation of the patient's ABO group requires confirmation of the red cell group by tests on the patient's serum (except for newborn infants).

Rh D grouping. Patient's red cells should be routinely tested with two different anti-D reagents, but without using an AHG technique which could lead to false positives. Where appropriate, reagent (diluent) controls with the patient's cells must be used to detect 'false' positive results due to reactions with the enhancing diluent.

Auto controls and D positive and negative specificity controls should be used (Appendix 1). Auto controls differ from reagent (diluent) controls in that the patient's serum is also included in the test.

It is not necessary to detect weak Rh D positive (D^u) in patients, as: (i) if the patient's Rh D group is doubtful, Rh D negative blood should be used; and (ii) women typed postnatally as Rh D negative, who are weak Rh D positive, will not be harmed by prophylactic IgG anti-D. However, it is important to detect weak D (high grade D^u) in the baby of an Rh D negative mother, as it may immunize the mother who should therefore receive prophylactic IgG anti-D. Anti-D reagents and techniques vary considerably in their ability to detect weak D. The indirect antiglobulin test is the most sensitive procedure, but selected anti-D reagents used by albumin (displacement) and enzyme techniques can detect high grade D^u. In the future the new generation of selected enhanced IgM monoclonal anti-D grouping reagents will reliably detect high grade D^u without the use of an antiglobulin test (Voak *et al.*, in preparation).

Antibody screening

Antibody screening tests provide an opportunity for early detection and identification of antibodies, thereby facilitating selection of suitable blood for the patient.

The patient's serum should be tested against at least two red cell suspensions, used separately and *not* pooled.

The screening cells must be group O and, as a minimum, should express the following antigens: C, c, D, E, e, M, N, S, s, P_1, K, k, Le^a, Le^b, Fy^a, Fy^b, Jk^a, Jk^b. At least one cell must be of the stronger D antigen combination R_2.

It is desirable to have antigens in the homozygous state, particularly for Jk^a, Jk^b, S, C, Fy^a, Fy^b, because red cells heterozygous for these antigens may fail to detect antibodies which would react positively with red cells homozygous for these antigens.

The antibody screening procedure is designed to detect antibodies of clinical significance. No single test will detect all the blood group antibodies, but an effective compromise is as follows.

1 Direct agglutination test with red cells suspended in NISS or LISS—recommended temperature 37°C to avoid detection of insignificant cold antibodies.

2 Indirect antiglobulin test (IAT) after incubation in NISS or LISS (Appendix 2).

Two-stage enzyme tests, although *not* mandatory, are recommended for antibody screening. Albumin displacement tests are also considered useful supportive techniques. However, both methods have their limitations and may fail to detect some antibodies reactive in a spin tube IAT. A one-stage enzyme mix test is not recommended (Scott *et al.*, 1988). However a phased mix test with a standardized enzyme based on the method of Odell *et al.* (1983) has been shown to be sensitive.

A positive result in the antibody screen must be followed by antibody identification against a comprehensive cell panel, which may require referral to a regional transfusion centre.

Group, antibody screen and save procedure

This is suitable for operative procedures where blood is usually not required but where it has been customary to have compatible blood on standby. It may be co-ordinated with maximum surgical blood ordering schedules for planned operations.

The patient's blood is ABO and Rh D grouped and screened for irregular antibodies; in the absence of irregular antibodies the serum is retained but no blood is cross-matched. When patients with a negative antibody screen require blood, cross-matching is carried out as in the section headed 'cross-matching' below.

This is a cost-effective strategy, which reduces the cross-match workload of the laboratory (Rock *et al.*, 1978; Haigh & Fairham, 1980) and should also lead to more effective usage of blood stocks.

Cross-matching

The standard compatibility procedure should include the direct cross-matching of the patient's serum with the donor red cells. These guidelines and the AABB Standards for Blood Banks and Transfusion Services (AABB, 1989) emphasize the importance of the donor–recipient cross-match as the ultimate check of ABO compatibility.

Methods that demonstrate ABO incompatibility and other clinically significant antibodies must be used. It is important to note that in addition to agglutination, haemolysis is a sign of incompatibility.

The actual procedure followed will depend on the clinical circumstances, since in emergency situations the sensitivity of the testing protocol may have to be relatively reduced in order to provide blood quickly for the patient.

ROUTINE CROSS-MATCHING

Select donor units for cross-matching on the basis of ABO and Rh D grouping and the antibody screen.

Test the patient's serum against donor red cells by:

Direct agglutination test. In NISS or LISS inspect for agglutination and haemolysis. The test can be read in the tube after gentle agitation over a x5 or 6 illuminated mirror, and incorporated with the indirect antiglobulin test as a one tube procedure.

Indirect antiglobulin test (IAT). Using a minimum incubation 15 minute LISS test or a 45 minute NISS test (Appendix 3) — the incubation temperature must be 37°C using a water bath or warmed block (air incubators are not recommended, but if used a longer incubation period of 60 minutes is required).

Alternative antiglobulin test procedures, should be validated and shown to be at least as sensitive as standard NISS or LISS methods before their routine use.

In this review of the guidelines the Working Party has addressed the contentious issue of the cross-match. The continuing unacceptable level of antibody detection failures in external proficiency trials (e.g. NEQAS for Blood Group Serology) dictates a cautious approach towards abbreviating the cross-match by omission of the antiglobulin phase. However, the consultant in charge of the blood bank may, after due consideration of the technical competence of the laboratory staff, decide to delete the AHG phase of the cross-match for patients who have a negative antibody screen and no previous record of irregular antibodies. This decision should be based on periodic assessment of individual staff competence by the simple, rapid procedure of 'blind' replicate antiglobulin tests with the proficiency standard anti-D (see Appendix 2 'Assessment of worker proficiency and correction of errors') which could be recorded as a 'certificate of competence' for each member of staff. Cell washing centrifuges must also be monitored regularly (see Appendix 3). These are essential prerequisites for abbreviating the routine cross-match to a rapid spin procedure.

EMERGENCY BLOOD ISSUE (WHERE TIME DOES NOT PERMIT FULL COMPATIBILITY TESTING)

An EDTA and a clotted sample should be obtained from the patient before the administration of intravenous colloids, such as Dextran and HES.

Patients should be ABO and Rh D grouped by rapid techniques and group-compatible blood issued. Exclude ABO incompatibility by a rapid spin cross-match (i.e. a spin agglutination test after 2–5 minute incubation at room temperature). Release the blood and convert the rapid spin test to a 15 min 37°C incubation phase for the IAT and/or do an antibody screen. Notify any incompatibility immediately.

If this procedure is followed, it should seldom be necessary to have to resort to group O Rh D negative blood. Should this need arise, only units which the blood bank has shown by confirmatory testing to be group O Rh D negative should be issued.

In the *massive transfusion* situation, where the number of units transfused in any 24 hour period exceeds the recipient's blood volume, compatibility testing may be reduced to checking the ABO/D groups of the transfused units.

After the emergency has been dealt with, retrospective antibody screening and/or cross-matching should be undertaken with the pretransfusion sample.

Donor units that have not been tested, or not fully tested, against the patient's serum should be clearly labelled, for example 'Selected for patient ...., but *not* cross-matched'.

Transfusion of infants less than 4 months old

Both baby and maternal blood samples should be ABO and Rh D grouped, the maternal serum screened for irregular antibodies, and a direct antiglobulin test (DAT) done on the baby's cells.

If a maternal antibody screen is negative and the baby's DAT is negative, blood of the same ABO and Rh D group as the infant may be issued without cross-matching, with the exception of infants of group O mothers (see below), even after repeated transfusions, provided the ABO and Rh D groups of the donor units are checked before issue. Recent studies indicate that infants under the age of 4 months do not make red cell alloantibodies even after multiple transfusions (Ludvigsen *et al.*, 1987). If maternal blood is not available, use the infant's serum for cross-matching in order to detect any maternal antibody that may have crossed the placenta.

Group A and B infants of group O mothers should be transfused with group O red cells. This is not necessary if the maternal serum is shown to contain only low titre IgG anti-A/B (i.e. < 32).

If the infant is suffering from HDN, or if irregular antibodies are detected in the maternal serum, it is important to use the maternal serum for compatibility testing. This may dictate the use of group O blood, and if the infant is not group O, care should be taken to ensure donor units have low titre anti-A and anti-B. If ABO haemolytic disease of the newborn (HDN) is suspected, group O blood of low titre anti-A and anti-B should be used.

Appendix 1: ABO and Rh D Grouping Controls

GENERAL REMARKS

Reagents should meet high potency specifications as laid down by UKBTS/NIBSC (1990) and ISBT/ICSH. (Engelfriet & Voak, 1987).

Before use, all new batches of reagents should be checked by showing that they give appropriate reactions with controls in the techniques used in the laboratory.

CONTROLS FOR ABO GROUPING

Each test or batch of tests on patient samples must also be controlled.

Anti-A: check for reactivity against A_2 cells, and for non-reactivity against B and O cells.

Anti-B: check for reactivity against B cells, and for non-reactivity against A_1 and O cells.

Anti-A,B: check for reactivity against A_2 and B cells, and for non-reactivity against O cells.

Inert AB serum (from the regional transfusion centre) and extra control cells may be used if thought appropriate. The use of monoclonal ABO typing reagents eliminates equivocal results caused by T activation of the patient's cells. If monoclonal reagents are *not* used, inert serum from group AB individuals could be used to check for polyagglutinability.

For the reverse ABO grouping of the patient's serum, the cells selected should be group A and B, and the patient's cells used as an auto control. Serum of infants is not suitable for reverse grouping.

CONTROLS FOR Rh D GROUPING

All anti-D reagents (IgG and IgM) should be checked for *specificity* with positive (O R_1r or O R_1R_2 cells), and negative controls (O r^1r or Orr). Additional controls to confirm the absorption of anti-A and anti-B (A_1rr and Brr cells) may be included to test each new batch of anti-D.

Tests using anti-D reagents should include parallel tests with *reagent (diluent) control* (as per manufacturer's instructions) to detect false positive results caused by reactions with the enhancing diluent. An *auto-control* should also be included to detect positive reactions due to *in vivo* sensitization. The auto control differs from the diluent control in that the patient's serum is included in the test. Monoclonal IgM anti-D reagents that are not potentiated do not require an additional auto-control as the ABO auto test also serves this function.

Appendix 2: The anti-human globulin (AHG) test: optimum conditions and quality control of the spin tube technique

In view of the high incidence of test failures found in International External Proficiency Trials, it is important to establish simple procedures for the detection and correction of errors in the spin tube AHG test (Engelfriet & Voak, 1987; Voak *et al.*, 1988). These recommendations are based on data from such trials and also the recent work of a joint working party of the International Committee for Standards in Haematology (ICSH) and the International Society of Blood Transfusion (ISBT), which has identified the main cause of false negatives in AHG tests as physical disruption of agglutination due to excessive agitation (shaking) at the reading stage of the test. However, reliable performance depends on the correct procedure at all stages of the test, and it was considered appropriate to make recommendations for the quality control of each stage of the spin tube AHG test (Voak *et al.*, 1988).

SENSITIZATION OF RED CELLS

Optimal sensitization of red cells is achieved by using the following serum : cell ratios.
1 For normal ionic saline solution (NISS) use at least 2 volumes (preferably 4 volumes) of serum to 1 volume of 3% washed red cells suspended in saline.
2 For low ionic saline solution (LISS) use 2 volumes of serum to 2 volumes of 1.5–2% red cells suspended in 0.033 mol LISS.
3 For low ionic strength additive solutions the manufacturer's instructions must be followed. NEQAS and the West of Scotland RTC proficiency testing scheme have both shown that LISS addition methods are less sensitive than LISS suspension methods.

The tubes should be shaken to mix the reactants, then incubated at 37°C (waterbath) for minimum incubation times of 45 minutes for NISS tests and 15 minutes for LISS tests.

WASHING THE RED CELLS FOR AHG TESTS

In practice, it is doubtful that maximum washing efficiency is ever achieved. Although in theory three washes is more than adequate, four washes are recommended because of the increased dilution of serum achieved. The essentials for efficient washing action are thorough mixing of the cells, followed by a vigorous injection of the saline wash to mix the cells and serum thoroughly throughout the tube, and then removal of as much of the supernatant as possible at the end of each washing cycle. Saline solutions produced commercially for *in vivo* irrigation/injection, and stored in plastic containers, should not be used for washing (Bruce *et al.*, 1986). The pH of saline or PBS solutions should not be less than pH 6 as this can lead to elution of some antibodies, for example anti-D.

To safeguard against inadequate washing that may occur with some cell washing centrifuges, it is recommended that 2 volumes of a potent AHG reagent per test should be used for spin tube methods (see Appendix 3). Machines that fail under these operating conditions should not be used.

SELECTION OF AHG REAGENTS

A suitable polyspecific AHG reagent (Engelfriet & Voak, 1987) should contain a potent anti-IgG and an adequate anti-complement reagent, for example anti-C3c (to detect *in vitro* cell-bound C3bi by complement fixing antibodies, for example anti-Lewis, anti-Kidd) and controlled levels of anti-C3d (to detect *in vivo* bound complement) or a satisfactory monoclonal anti-C3d that gives equivalent sensitivity (e.g. BRIC-8).

A coloured dye (usually green) added to the AHG reagent by the manufacturer enables the operator to observe that AHG has been added to each test.

OPTIMUM CENTRIFUGATION AND READING PROCEDURE

Various RCF and times (seconds) satisfactory for spin-tube tests are as follows:

RCF (g)	110	200–220	500	1000
Time (seconds)	60	25–30	15	8–10

For reading the results a shake-tube technique generally gives lower grades of agglutination than other reading techniques. Only the strongest complete (C) grade of agglutination seems able to withstand a shake procedure without some degree of disruption. It is therefore recommended that a gentle agitation or tip-and-roll method or the microscopic examination of reactants transferred by pipette on to a slide are the optimum reading procedures in the spin-tube AHG test. While it is not the intention of this chapter to recommend microscope reading of all tests, as it is accepted that reactions read with cells in the tube over a x5 or x6 illuminated mirror should have adequate sensitivity for routine work, macroscopic reading of the test by the naked eye is *not* adequate.

QUALITY CONTROL OF EACH BATCH OF AHG TESTS

The routine quality control of the potency of the AHG reagent should be evaluated by a separate positive control test, i.e. a low affinity IgG anti-D, for example BCSH proficiency standard anti-D, diluted to about 0.1–0.2 IU/ml to give a 1 + /2 + reaction with a pool of four Rh D positive red cells.

The positive control using red cells weakly sensitized with anti-D is intended to demonstrate whether the washed cells are still contaminated with human immunoglobulin for whatever reason, and that the AHG reagent is still potent. A failure in the control test makes it essential to retest the whole batch of tests. This weak indicator system is more sensitive to partial neutralization of the AHG reagent than the frequently used procedure of adding strongly sensitized cells to all negative AHG tests. The same batch of saline/PBS must be used to wash the batch of tests and the controls, thus demonstrating that the washing solution is free from contamination with serum immunoglobulins.

VALIDATION OF THE WHOLE AHG TEST PROCEDURE

This is achieved by a combination of quality control procedures.

1 Cleaning and maintenance schedules of cell washing machines, as per a machine cleaning SOP (see Appendix 3).
   (a) Wash the machine thoroughly with distilled water at the end of each day.
   (b) Soak all machine tubing in hypochlorite solution once weekly then wash thoroughly.
   (c) Evaluate the cell washing centrifuges weekly by replicate tests to demonstrate any washing inefficiencies (see p. 162).

2 Initial and periodic evaluation of worker reading skills by replicate tests to eliminate false negative errors due to excessive agitation in the reading technique.

3 The use of a weak positive control with each batch of tests. A negative control may be used but is not essential as most tests are negative.

4 Use of coloured AHG reagents to enable the operator to observe that AHG reagent has been added to each test.

5 The addition of AHG control sensitized cells to all negative tests. This latter procedure effectively demonstrates serum contamination of antiglobulin tests at levels greater than 1 in 1500. However, the use of strongly sensitized cells gives an illusion of safety (Voak *et al.*, 1986; 1988) for example: in a recent NEQAS exercise it was found that 6% of participants missed 0.3 IU/ml (2 + /3 +) anti-D and 41% of participants missed 0.1 IU/ml (1 + /2 +) anti-D in AHG tests with R_1r cells. The use of control cells by 68.5% of the participants did not reveal any of these false negative errors suggesting that strong control cells reacted normally in these false negative tests.

The production of satisfactory AHG control cells can be achieved by limiting the level of anti-D sensitization to that which gives a negative test in the presence of 1 in 1000 parts serum in saline (Appendix 4).

ASSESSMENT OF WORKER PROFICIENCY AND CORRECTION OF ERRORS (Voak *et al.*, 1986; 1988)

It is recommended that all staff (including on-call staff who do not routinely work in the blood bank) should be assessed with 'blind' replicate antiglobulin tests using a BCSH Proficiency Standard Anti-D* (0.1–0.2 IU/ml) giving relatively weak 1+/2+ macroscopic agglutination to assess their competence to perform AHG tests. This is a rapid procedure of staff evaluation which should be carried out periodically.

Details of the procedure are as follows.

1 A batch of sensitized cells is prepared by incubating 16 ml of the BCSH proficiency standard anti-D at the recommended dilution with 8 ml of 3–5% washed R_1r or R_1R_2 red cells. These sensitized cells should give a 1+/2+ reaction by a spin tube IAT.

2 Twelve tubes are labelled for blind tests by another person. One volume of 3% 1+/2+ sensitized cells and 2 volumes of group AB inert serum (to simulate the volumes of serum used in routine tests) are placed in 9 random tubes, and then 1 volume of unsensitized cells + 2 volumes of group AB inert serum placed in the remaining tubes. The position of the various tests is recorded.

3 The tests are washed thoroughly four times, AHG added and the tests spun and read.

4 The number of false negative (and false positive) results are recorded for each worker and analysed in relation to reading and/or washing technique.

It is advisable to give immediate tuition to any workers who have shown washing or reading test faults, followed by further blind replicate tests to demonstrate improvement and to restore confidence.

Appendix 3: Quality control of cell washing centrifuges (Voak *et al.*, 1986; 1988)

The procedures described relate to the use of cell washing centrifuges in the spin tube AHG test. The machines should not be used for washing whole blood samples for other serological procedures.

New machines

Machines should only be accepted after they have been installed and adjusted by the agent's representative, and their washing efficiency proved by three machine loads of replicate tests with 1+/2+ sensitized cells as in Appendix 2. The centrifuge should

*Supplied through the National Institute for Biological Standards and Quality Control (NIBSC) at a nominal charge.

conform to the mechanical containment requirements of BS 4402 (BSI, 1982) and *Electrical Safety Codes for Hospital Laboratory Equipment* (DHSS, 1986–7).

Procedure with all machines

1 Tubes must conform to manufacturer's recommendations. Glass tubes are recommended as cell buttons are far more difficult to dislodge from plastic tubes and IgG bound to plastic tubes has been found to inhibit anti-IgG (Black & Kay, 1986). Optimal tube length is 75 mm; overlong tubes have been found to cause inadequate washing in several makes of machines through the tube lip making contact with the saline wash port and preventing the correct volume of saline entering the tube.
2 Use four wash cycles with 3 ml (or more) of saline; check that these volumes are correct.
3 Use 2 volumes of an AHG reagent suitable for the spin tube technique.
4 In the final spin phase determine the spin time and RCF combination for the machine that will give optimal sensitivity with freedom from false positive reactions.
5 Clean the cell washing centrifuges daily to avoid a build-up of serum contamination that may cause back contamination of tests from droplets created by the turbulence of the moving components of the machine.
6 Routine check of the washing efficiency at least once a week (at random) by at least one machine-load of replicate tests with 1 + /2 + sensitized cells, as in Appendix 2.

The number of failures for each machine is recorded. A failure is a test that gives a reaction less than the expected 1 + /2 + result.

7 Action to be taken with faulty centrifuge washers:
(a) withdraw machine from routine use for servicing;
(b) notify important faults to the manufacturer and the Department of Health, Supplies Technology Division. This information will assist manufacturers to improve the specification of machines.

Appendix 4: Quality control of AHG control cells for addition to negative tests

PROCEDURE

1 Prepare two tubes (10 × 75 mm) with one volume of 3% unsensitized cells; wash four times.
2 Add two volumes of AHG to each of the tubes, mix well, spin and read the tubes to confirm the tests are negative.
3 Add one volume of 1 in 1000 serum in saline to one tube and one volume of saline as a control to the other tube and incubate for 1 minute at RT.
4 Add one volume of AHG control cells to each tube, mix, spin and read the tests.

A test containing the 1 in 1000 serum in saline should be negative and the control tube should give at least a 2 + level of reaction. Note that the direct test with AHG on the AHG control cells will be a strong 3 + /C, but in the 'down grade' reaction in a washed negative antiglobulin test the reaction will be reduced to a 2 + /3 + reaction by pooled cell effects.

References

AABB (1989) *Standards for Blood Banks and Transfusion Services* 13th edn. American Association of Blood Banks, Arlington, Virginia.

BSCH (1987) Guidelines for compatibility testing in hospital blood banks. *Clinical and Laboratory Haematology* **9**, 333–341.

Black D. & Kay J. (1986) Influence of tube type on the antiglobulin test. *Medical Laboratory Sciences* **43**, 169–173.

BSI (1982) *Safety Requirements for Laboratory Centrifuges*. British Standards Institution, BS 4402.

Bruce M., Watt A.H., Hare W., Blue A. & Mitchell R. (1986) A serious source of error in antiglobulin testing. *Transfusion* **26**, 177–181.

DHSS (1986–7) *Electrical safety code for hospital laboratory equipment II—HE1 158, 165*. Department of Health and Social Security, Scientific and Technical Branch, Russell Square, London.

Engelfriet C.P. & Voak D. (1987) International reference polyspecific anti-human globulin reagents. *Vox Sanguinis* **53**, 241–247.

Haigh T. & Fairham S.A. (1980) Advantages of low ionic strength saline (LISS) techniques in blood bank management. *Medical Laboratory Sciences* **37**, 119–125.

Ludvigsen C.W., Swanson J.J., Thompson T.R. & McCullough J. (1987) The failure of neonates to form red blood cell alloantibodies in response to multiple transfusion. *American Journal of Clinical Pathology* **87**, 250–251.

Odell W.R., Roxby D.J., Ryall R.G. & Seshaadri R.S. (1983) A LISS spin-enzyme method for the detection of red cell antibodies and its use in routine antibody screen procedures. *Transfusion* **23**, 373–376.

Rock G., Baxter A., Charron M. & Jhaveri J. LISS—an effective way to increase blood utilisation. *Transfusion* **18**, 228–232.

Scott M.L., Voak D. & Downie D.M. (1988) Optimum enzyme activity and a new technique for antibody detection: an explanation for the poor performance of the one-stage mix technique. *Medical Laboratory Sciences* **45**, 7–18.

UKBTS/NIBSC (1990) Guidelines for the Blood Transfusion Services in the United Kingdom. Vol. III *Guidelines for reagents for Blood Group Serology and HLA Typing*. HMSO, London.

Voak D., Downie D.M., Moore B.P.L., Ford D.S., Engelfriet C.P. & Case J. (1986) Quality control of anti-human globulin tests: use of replicate tests to improve performance. *Biotest Bulletin* **1**, 41–52.

Voak D., Downie D.M., Moore B.P.L., Ford D.S., Engelfriet C.P. & Case J. (1988) Replicate tests for the detection and correction of errors in anti-human globulin (AHG) tests: optimum conditions and quality control. *Haematologia* **21**, 3–16.

Voak D., Downie D.M., Sonneborne H.H., Ernst M., Davies D., Van Rhenen D.J. & Overbeeke M. Donor Rh D typing without an antiglobulin test for weak D (D^u). Reagent development and quality assurance. (In preparation).

15 Microplate Techniques in Liquid Phase Blood Grouping and Antibody Screening

Prepared by the
Blood Transfusion Task Force

This chapter is an introduction to microplate serology prepared at a time of very active research and development. Antibody detection techniques are expected to improve during the lifetime of this publication.

Approximately 25% of hospital blood banks are ABO and D grouping by microplate techniques. These procedures are being adequately performed by various automated, semi-automated or manual test systems.

Antibody screening by microplate techniques is only being carried out by a small percentage of hospital blood banks but there is likely to be a change to antiglobulin tests by microplate procedures as soon as the methods have been thoroughly tested and approved. The antiglobulin test procedure presented in these guidelines is a liquid-phase antiglobulin test and there are one or two weak links in the procedure which could give rise to serious errors.

1 Antiglobulin reagents standardized for spin-tube tests may be subject to prozones in liquid phase microplate tests. Each new batch of antiglobulin reagent must be standardized by the microplate procedure in use to show that the reagent is at its optimum anti-IgG dilution for use. However dilutions greater than 1 : 2 may seriously compromise the anti-complement activity of the reagent.

2 Automated cell washers for microplates are currently under development and should be evaluated by replicate tests with weak anti-D sensitized cells. Studies so far have shown that machines may not be as good as manual procedures for the removal of supernatant and the mixing of cells during the wash phase.

3 The combination of diluted anti-IgG and poor washing procedures may lead to neutralization of anti-IgG and cause false negative errors.

Future development for improved antiglobulin tests in microplates by a solid phase system is now well advanced and workers proposing to change to antibody screening by microplates are advised to bear this in mind.

It is hoped that microplate methodology will move towards standardization based on national guidelines using standard antibody reagents for the validation of new microplate procedures.

Introduction

The 96-well microplate format which is in routine use in many blood banks today was first used in viral serological investigations (Sever, 1962). Wegmann and Smithies (1966; 1968) described a technique using V-well microplates and 0.03% red cell suspensions for saline, enzyme and antiglobulin methods in blood group serology. Subsequent publications (Crawford *et al.*, 1970; Warlow & Tills, 1978; Parker *et al.*, 1978) confirmed the versatility of the system which could be used with a wide range of volumes and concentrations of reagents in U- and V-well plates.

In 1984 two groups of workers described the automated interpretation of ABO and Rh grouping tests in microplates (Bowley *et al.*, 1984; Severns *et al.*, 1984).

The advantages of microplates which workers in many blood transfusion laboratories have identified may be summarized as follows.

1 Some specialist techniques allow small volumes and low concentrations of sera and red cells to be used; any reduced requirement for reagents can lead to substantial cost savings. In general the sensitivity of microplate techniques increases as the cell concentration decreases.

2 Batching of samples has become much more common in hospital blood banks and this can be achieved in microplates with a considerable economy in laboratory space and staff time.

3 Automated microplate systems have enabled many blood banks to utilize the many advantages of on-line data capture previously available only to very large laboratories. These advantages include: reduction in reading and transcription errors; savings in staff time; the use of bar codes for sample and microplate identification; and integration into a comprehensive computer system for pathology data.

4 Larger laboratories can benefit from several items of microplate hardware which may reduce operator time even further (reagent dispensers, sample handlers and cell washers for example).

There are however a number of important practical points which need to be considered.

1 Microplate techniques using higher cell concentrations (2–3%) are recommended in this chapter because of ease of reading both visually and in automated systems. These routine techniques may not provide substantial savings in reagent costs compared with conventional tube techniques.

2 The scope for economies in small blood banks will clearly be less. However, the cost of microplate hardware and disposables is reasonable and should not preclude their use in these laboratories.

3 Microplate technology has not progressed to the point where sensitive antibody screening techniques are available for automated determination in the routine laboratory. In addition, as with conventional tube techniques, it should be remembered that antibody screening in microplates requires considerable technical expertise.

4 Product liability for a reagent will pass from the manufacturer to the user if the manufacturer's instructions are not followed exactly (Doughty, 1989). Most reagents are not available already standardized for microplate use and therefore the onus is on the user to ensure that they perform satisfactorily in the technique to be used. Guidelines are given in Appendix 6 for standardizing reagents for routine use, and in Appendix 8 for validating a new technique by comparison with an established technique. When these tests are performed they should be performed in accordance with a written Standard Operating Procedure (SOP) (see Chapter 19). The batch numbers, details of the methodology including incubation times and temperature, and the results obtained should be accurately recorded and these records kept. The results should be reviewed and signed by a nominated quality assurance (QA) officer or senior scientist before using the reagent routinely. If diluted reagents are to be stored it should be shown and documented that there is no loss of activity during the assigned storage period (see Appendix 6).

The shape of the wells in 96-well microplates is usually described by manufacturers as 'U-well', 'V-well' or 'flat bottomed'. Flat bottomed plates are useful in ELISA technology but are unsuitable for liquid-phase blood group serology. Saline, enzyme and antiglobulin serological techniques can be performed in U- and V-well plates. U-well plates are preferred to V-well plates for resuspension techniques because of the ease of resuspension of red cells prior to reading and because of their superior optical quality when using some automated plate readers. Resuspension techniques for ABO and D grouping are rapid and simple in manual serology and they are essential in automated serology as adequate photometric discrimination between positive and negative reactions can only be achieved with currently available plate readers when red cells in negative reactions are fully resuspended. The loss of sensitivity using a resuspension technique is acceptable in blood grouping provided that properly standardized reagent antisera are used; enzyme treatment of red cells will also improve reaction strength. Only a resuspension technique in U-well plates has been recommended in this document (p. 174) for ABO and D grouping.

A full discussion of the relative merits of U- and V-well plates for antibody screening is to be found on pp. 177–8.

Although microplate techniques have been available to blood group serologists for almost 3 decades, they have only gained widespread popularity in the UK during the last 5 years, probably because of increasing workloads in blood transfusion laboratories and the recent availability of packaged automated systems. Solid phase techniques and image analysis systems are being researched in several laboratories and this rapid development in technology constitutes a major difficulty when preparing a document such as this. The aim of this document is to give basic guidelines in blood grouping and antibody screening in microplates for transfusion laboratories handling routine specimens. Liquid phase techniques only are dealt with as these have been shown to be consistently reliable for blood grouping and antibody screening and because a wide range of hardware is available to suit the requirements of most laboratories. General guidelines for pretransfusion testing are to be found in Chapter 14.

Equipment

Microplates

Untreated rigid polystyrene microplates should be purchased because polyvinyl chloride and polystyrene plates treated for solid phase ELISA have a greater protein-binding capacity which is not desirable in liquid phase serology. Either new or used plates are suitable. If reusing plates, these must first be soaked in a mild detergent, rinsed thoroughly with a final rinse in distilled water and allowed to dry face down at room temperature or at 37°C. Alternatively, an ultrasonic bath may be used for cleaning. Before use they should be examined and plates which are scored or otherwise damaged discarded. Static is sometimes a problem when using new plates but only rarely so when using concentrations of red cells greater than 1% (see p. 173). Pretreatment of plates with albumin and/or Tween is not necessary for ABO and D grouping techniques described below but may be necessary for anti human globulin (AHG) testing (see pp. 173 & 178).

The characteristics of microplates (of a given product code) from a single manufacturer may reasonably be assumed to be consistent, although it should be noted that distributors may change their sources of supply. A batch of tests should consist of microplates from a single manufacturer (see p. 181).

Pipettes

Pasteur pipettes delivering drops of approximately 30–35 μl of liquid are suitable for routine blood grouping. When used for pipetting antisera, one pasteur pipette should be used for each antiserum and then discarded. When used for pipetting serum, plasma, or red cells from a specimen of blood, the pipette must be washed thoroughly in at least five changes of clean saline. Pipettes with similar delivery volumes should be used in each batch of tests.

Hand-held and automated single-channel or multi-channel dispensers are suitable for microplate use. Variable volume dispensers covering the range 20–50 μl will be found to be most useful.

Manufacturers' reagent droppers may deliver up to 50 μl of liquid and this must be taken into account when dispensing these reagents. Consistent volumes of serum and cells must be used in all routine and quality control procedures (see p. 181).

Centrifuges

Centrifuge heads for carrying microplates are available for most bench-top centrifuges. Centrifuges with a rotor radius of less than 15 cm are adequate for resuspension techniques but are not suitable for streaming (trailing) techniques as centrifugation leads to uneven settling patterns, with cell buttons displaced to the side in peripheral wells. Floor standing centrifuges may be inconvenient in routine use as deceleration times are prolonged. When using rotors which allow stacking of plates, a trial should be carried out on each make of microplates in use to ascertain whether the plates are damaged during centrifugation.

Recommended centrifugation conditions are discussed in the appropriate sections. Centrifugation should be sufficient to sediment the cells prior to reading but in both U-well (resuspension) and V-well (streaming) techniques over-centrifugation can lead to difficulties: the necessary vigorous resuspension in U-wells may lead to increased fragmentation of agglutinates while in V-wells streaming times may be increased to an unacceptable level.

Microplate shakers

These are available from several manufacturers. They are recommended for mixing serum and cells before incubation, and are essential for resuspension techniques in U-well plates. In antiglobulin testing they are useful for resuspending red cells prior to addition of wash fluid and for mixing after addition of antiglobulin reagent. Two-place shakers are preferred as four-place shakers may give uneven agitation. Variable speed shakers are useful but a trial should be carried out with these to determine the maximum speed which can be used that does not lead to splashing and cross-contamination between wells; this will depend on the volume of fluid in each well.

In resuspension techniques agitation of red cells prior to reading must be sufficient to resuspend cells fully in negative reactions, but should also be kept to a minimum in order to limit the disruption of agglutinates. It is therefore recommended (see pp. 175 & 179) that agitation in these techniques should be continued to the point where all negative control reactions are just fully resuspended.

Reading aids

These are recommended for routine use, and will enable interpretation of weak positive results to be made. For U-well (resuspension) techniques, reading is best accomplished while the plate is horizontal, reading from below using a magnifying mirror or from above over a light box with a diffuse screen. Specially constructed magnifying mirrors are available from several suppliers of microplate equipment.

Automated plate readers

Most automated plate readers are based on ELISA reading systems. Principles of operation, limitations of use and software versatility vary considerably between systems. A discussion of these is outside the scope of this chapter but helpful information can be obtained from manufacturers or distributors. Manufacturers' instructions for the use and maintenance of the equipment should be followed.

The difference in optical density at the wavelength in use between red cells and supernatant fluid must be as great as possible in automated systems because this gives the greatest discrimination between positive and negative reactions. In blood grouping the presence of reagent dyes or traces of haemolysis in test red cells may reduce this discrimination. Similarly in reverse grouping the presence of haemoglobin, bilirubin or lipids in the test serum may also adversely affect interpretation. As a general rule ELISA readers will give the best discrimination in routine use when a wavelength of approximately 540 nm is used.

Reagents

Blood specimens

Blood samples should be as fresh as possible for blood grouping. Venous blood should be drawn into a clean container and stored preferably refrigerated at 4°C if not tested within 12 hours. Clotted blood may be used but it may be difficult to obtain sufficient free red cells from some samples. Anticoagulated blood is convenient for blood grouping in microplates but the use of plasma, especially from citrated samples, may lead to the non-detection of weak or complement binding antibodies.

Antisera

At present antisera standardized for use by the techniques described on pages 175 and 180 are not generally available and so each laboratory should ensure that antisera are specific, sufficiently potent and otherwise suitable for microplate use. All reagents which need to be restandardized for microplate use should be tested for potency and specificity as described in Appendix 6. All reagents should be tested prior to routine use as described in Appendix 7. Appropriate documentation of these tests should be maintained as discussed on pages 165 and 181.

BLOOD GROUPING ANTISERA

In general, antisera with a bovine serum albumin (BSA) concentration between 1 and 7% should be used. High concentrations of proteins or polymers such as ficoll, PVP or dextran cause red cells to stick to the surface of the wells, leading to difficulty in resuspension of red cells in blood grouping work. Additives in antisera may also alter the position of the meniscus of the reaction mixture and hence its optical properties and this is clearly very important when using an automated reading system. Monolayering of red cells may occur when using antisera with too low a protein concentration, for example when using reagents highly diluted in saline, and this may also cause problems in interpretation (see p. 173).

Many blood grouping reagents can be diluted for use in microplates but the choice of diluent will depend on the composition of that reagent, especially the presence of additives, and on the antibody potency. Most ABO and monoclonal IgM anti-D reagents will give excellent results when used undiluted but may give equally good reactions when diluted in phosphate buffered saline (PBS) (see Appendix 1) containing 1–3% bovine serum albumin (BSA). Chemically modified D-grouping reagents sometimes contain additives in high enough concentration to cause problems when used undiluted, but dilution in PBS or in 1% BSA in PBS may improve reaction patterns while maintaining an adequate antibody potency. Polyclonal anti-D sera suitable for slide and rapid tube use are usually unsuitable for microplate use if undiluted because of the high concentration of additives but may be useable when diluted in PBS or 1% BSA in PBS. The intensity of dye in coloured reagents may also cause problems in interpretation in manual and automated microplate techniques and dilution of the reagent may be helpful.

POLYSPECIFIC ANTIGLOBULIN REAGENTS

Polyspecific antiglobulin (AHG) reagents which are standardized for microplate testing are not yet widely available. Antiglobulin reagents which have been standardized for the spin tube technique can be used but it should be noted that some reagents do not give reliable results if used undiluted as the rate of red cell streaming is retarded. An additional problem is that the level of anti-IgG in the reagent may not be optimal for microplate techniques, leading to prozones being encountered with weakly sensitized cells. These problems may be overcome by diluting the reagent between 1 + 1 and 1 + 7 in 1% BSA in PBS, but the potency of the reagent must be assured to be adequate as described in Appendix 6. If a polyspecific reagent is used both the anti-IgG and anti-complement activity should be assessed. It is important that polyspecific and anti-IgG reagents are diluted as little as possible (less than 1 + 7) because diluted reagents are more easily neutralized by any residual serum and adequate washing of cells may not be consistently achievable under these circumstances. This may be demonstrated by a quality control procedure using replicate tests (see p. 181).

Dyed antiglobulin reagents do not usually cause problems in interpretation of results.

BOVINE SERUM ALBUMIN (BSA) FOR USE AS A DILUENT

Different batches of BSA may have very different properties and this must be borne in mind when diluting reagents. For example, both the degree of potentiation of a reaction and the ability of red cells to be resuspended for reading may be affected by the presence and nature of polymers. Some preparations of BSA contain antibodies which react with enzyme treated red cells. BSA used for dilution of antiglobulin reagents must be essentially free of IgG. A single batch of BSA should be used when standardizing a reagent for microplate use as described in Appendix 6.

Reagent red cells and red cell diluents

PBS, LISS and preservative (modified Alsever's) solutions which are used for suspending red cells in tube techniques may also be used in microplate techniques. However, enzyme techniques are commonly used in microplate blood grouping because the forces involved in resuspending negative reactions in the resuspension technique may lead to fragmentation of weak agglutinates. The choice of which diluent to use will depend upon a number of factors.

TEST RED CELLS FOR BLOOD GROUPING

Potent monoclonal IgM ABO and D grouping reagents can often be used successfully with test red cells suspended in PBS or LISS. When standardizing these antisera (see Appendix 6) it may be found that certain weak phenotypes react poorly and under these circumstances the one-stage bromelain method described in Appendix 5 is likely to give better results. Note that one-stage enzyme techniques may also reduce the serological activity of an antiserum (particularly monoclonal reagents) and so the incubation time of antiserum with cells should be carefully controlled during standardization and quality assessment and recorded in the appropriate documentation. The use of a bromelain diluent may also allow greater dilution of reagents. If a polyclonal IgG anti-D reagent is used then a bromelain method will be the technique of choice. Cells used to control ABO and D grouping antisera should be suspended in the same diluent as test cells.

Well-packed red cells need not normally be washed prior to resuspension in a suitable diluent for blood grouping. Residual serum or plasma in cell suspensions should be limited as far as possible as rouleaux or inhibition of the antibody–antigen reaction may otherwise be encountered when grouping blood samples of some patients. If packed cells are not available, as may be the case with clotted specimens, it is recommended that the red cells are washed once before use.

REAGENT RED CELLS FOR REVERSE (SERUM) BLOOD GROUPING

Reverse ABO grouping may be carried out using cells suspended in PBS or LISS. The reactions obtained in the resuspension method (see p. 175) are normally adequate for visual or automated interpretation. However some sera (for example from elderly people and patients with haematological conditions) may give weak reactions and under these circumstances, or as a routine practice, the method for reverse grouping can be amended as follows:

1 increase the serum : cell ratio by a factor of 2 (i.e. use two drops of serum and one drop of 3% reagent cells); and/or

2 ensure that the incubation temperature is kept at 20°C or below; or

3 use enzyme treated cells. This will potentiate the reverse grouping reactions substantially but may be associated with the detection of enzyme dependent panagglutinins and cold reactive antibodies of no clinical importance.

If a non-enzyme method is used, red cells supplied as a 3% suspension in a preservative medium may be used directly. Cell suspensions prepared in the laboratory should be made from blood either freshly obtained or from blood stored aseptically for not more than 3 weeks in an anticoagulant such as CPD or CPDA-1. These cells should be washed and resuspended to 3% in PBS or LISS and discarded within 24 hours or before if haemolysis is evident.

EDTA should be added to reagent cell diluents to prevent haemolysis (see Appendix 2). This is particularly important when using automated plate readers as haemolysis may be incorrectly interpreted as a negative reaction. Appendix 4 gives a suitable (2 stage) method for enzyme treatment of reagent cells.

REAGENT RED CELLS FOR ANTIBODY SCREENING

Much the same considerations apply regarding selection of reagent cell diluent (PBS or LISS) as when using conventional tube techniques and this is dealt with more fully in Chapter 14. Reagent cells supplied in preservative solutions may be used directly or in-house red cell preparations made as discussed on p. 172.

Techniques using reagent cell concentrations less than 3% may give improved sensitivity for antibody screening and this is discussed in pp. 177 and 178.

Autologous (auto), diluent and AB serum controls

With all red cell grouping techniques it is essential to ensure that the cells are not agglutinated (or aggregated) except when the desired antibody–antigen reaction has taken place. Red cells which have been coated *in vivo* with antibody (i.e. have a positive direct antiglobulin test) may show 'false' positive reactions when potentiators are used in the red cell diluent (e.g. enzymes) or in the antiserum diluent (e.g. albumin, ficoll, dextran). Even if the cells being typed have a negative direct antiglobulin test, such potentiators can sometimes cause difficulties in microplate techniques.

If an antiserum is supplied with a reagent diluent control ('diluent control') then that must be used in parallel with the antiserum for all cells tested. If no such diluent control is available then the manufacturer's guidelines should be followed but in the absence of guidance, AB serum, 5% BSA in PBS or autologous serum or plasma should be used. If diluted typing reagents are used the working diluent control should consist of AB serum or the manufacturer's diluent control diluted in the same diluent and to the same degree as the least dilute antiserum used. The working diluent control should therefore contain the highest concentration of protein or other macromolecules to be found in any of the reagents used.

Problems with static and non-specific binding

Occasionally it is found that during pipetting serum or cell suspensions into a microplate there is a tendency for the drop to be pulled towards the side of the well, making accurate pipetting impossible. This is caused by the build-up of static electric charges on polystyrene plates. Some workers and environments seem to be more prone to static problems than others. One of the following remedies should prove effective:

1 stand the microplate on a damp cloth;
2 use an anti-static gun;
3 ensure that any adhesive cover is removed at least 15 minutes prior to using the plate.

Another problem is encountered during antiglobulin testing when monolayering of red cells may occur during the incubation or washing stages of the test. This monolayering may occur because of static charges or because of non-specific binding of immunoglobulin. Monolayering problems can usually be resolved by rinsing the microplate in distilled water containing photographic wetting agent or 0.02% Tween 20 before use and by using PBS containing 0.1% BSA and 0.02% Tween 20 for the wash solution. When using very low concentrations (less than 0.2%) of cells pretreatment of the plate with albumin may be necessary. This may be achieved by filling each well with water containing 0.5% BSA and incubating for 1 hour at 37°C or overnight at 4°C. The plate is then washed in water with the final rinse containing photographic wetting agent.

Methodology for ABO and D grouping

Minimum requirements

The patient's red cells should be tested using at least one example of each of anti-A and anti-B and two examples of anti-D. The patient's serum or plasma should be tested with A cells and B cells. The patient's red cells should also be tested with the patient's serum or plasma (auto control) or with a diluent or AB serum control (see p. 173).

Each batch of tests should be tested with cells which control all the antisera used on the plate. It is recommended (see Chapter 14) that the following cells are used to control ABO and D grouping reagents:

Anti-A A_2, B and O cells;
Anti-B A_1, B and O cells;
Anti-A,B A_2, B and O cells;
Anti-D O R_1r, and O r′r or O rr cells.

If a bromelain diluent is used to augment the reactions with ABO and D grouping reagents (see p. 171) then it is recommended that the efficacy of this diluent is controlled for each batch of tests by testing D positive cells suspended in this diluent with a weak anti-D serum (final concentration 0.25 IU/ml or less and made from a source material containing 10 IU/ml or less of anti-D) and with AB (inert) serum using the method employed for routine ABO and D grouping.

These controls must give the correct reaction patterns otherwise the results of that batch of tests are invalidated.

Layout

The layout of sera and cells in the microplate must be described in a laboratory Standard Operating Procedure (SOP) (see also p. 181).

Recommended U-well (resuspension) technique

1 Prepare a 3% suspension of reagent red cells in a suitable diluent (see p. 172 and Appendix 4).

2 Prepare a 3% suspension of test red cells in a suitable diluent (see p. 171 and Appendix 5).
3 Add one drop (see p. 167) of antiserum to the appropriate wells of a U-well plate.
4 Add one drop of diluent control to the appropriate wells (if required).
5 Add one or two drops of test serum or plasma to the appropriate wells for serum (reverse) grouping and for auto controls (if required).
6 Add one drop of a 3% suspension of test cells to the appropriate wells containing antiserum, and diluent or auto controls.
7 Add one drop of a 3% suspension of reagent red cells to the appropriate wells containing test serum or plasma for reverse grouping.
8 Agitate the plate to mix the reactants, preferably with a microplate shaker, taking care to ensure that no contamination occurs between wells.
9 Leave the plate at ambient temperature for 15 minutes and centrifuge at 100 g for 40 seconds (or suitable alternative rcf and time).
10 Resuspend the red cells using a microplate shaker. The time of agitation will depend upon the speed and orbit of mixing. *Over-agitation will reduce the strength of agglutination* and this can be avoided by switching off the microplate shaker as soon as a known negative reaction (for example a diluent control) is fully resuspended and positive reactions dislodged. This observable process requires expertise which has to be acquired by practice. Each batch of tests (see pp. 174 and 181) set up must contain control cells and these must show correct reaction patterns.
11 Typical reaction patterns are shown in Figure 15.1. These may be interpreted visually (see p. 169) or using an automated or semi-automated system, set up and operated in accordance with the manufacturer's specifications.

Predispensed plates

One of the advantages of using microplates for blood grouping is that a large batch of plates may be dispensed with antisera (and reagent red cells for reverse grouping). A multi-channel pipette or automated microplate dispenser may be used which can save considerable time, but in these circumstances particular care must be taken to ensure that contamination between reagents does not take place. Static may be more troublesome when using an automated dispenser: ways of avoiding static are dealt with on p. 173. The use of dyed reagents allows a visual check on the addition of antisera to plates. Predispensed plates should be kept covered at 4°C until required in a place where they are not likely to be accidentally disturbed. Microplate lids and adhesive covers are available commercially. Particular care in labelling predispensed microplates is needed to ensure that reagents can be correctly identified by all workers in the laboratory.

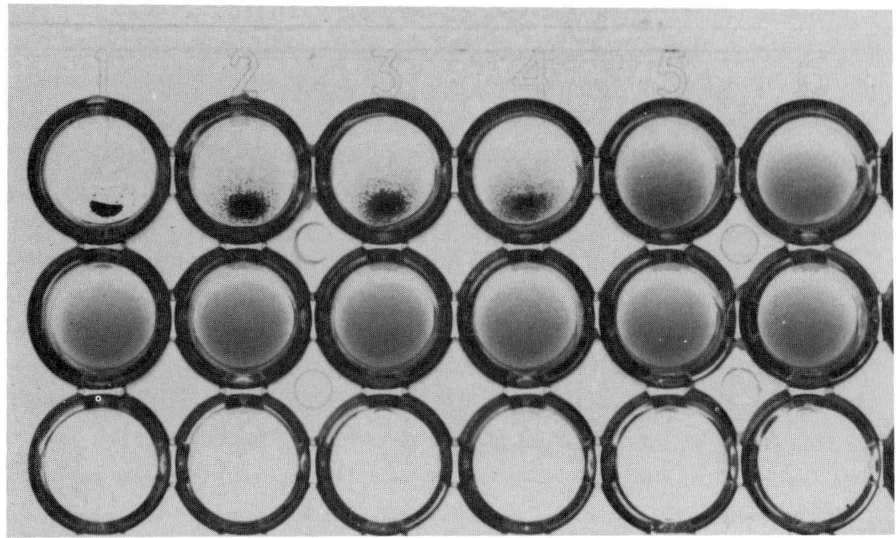

Fig. 15.1 Reaction patterns in a U-well resuspension technique. Top row, left to right: a strongly positive result followed by successively weaker reactions. Second row: negative reactions.

It is recommended that in order to avoid evaporation of reagents predispensed microplates should not be stored for more than 24 hours at 4°C. Predispensed plates should not be stored longer than this or frozen unless acceptable limits of storage temperature and shelf life are determined (see Appendix 6). Freezing and thawing of diluted antisera is likely to result in loss of activity. This may be minimized by freezing and thawing rapidly once only.

Methodology for antibody screening

General comments

Guidelines for the selection of cells are given elsewhere (Chapter 14).

Manual polybrene and albumin displacement techniques can be performed in microplates but are not convenient in the context of antibody screening. Enzyme and antiglobulin techniques are recommended for antibody screening and these are further discussed below. Antibody identification can be done by the same techniques as described below, but substituting the screening cells with a panel of cells.

Prewarming test serum and screening cells to 37°C will reduce the incidence of unwanted positive results caused by clinically non-significant antibodies with a low thermal range. In addition, incubation at 37°C should be performed in a warm air incubator, with plates stacked not more than two high.

Each plate of enzyme and antiglobulin tests should carry a weak positive control, for example a weak anti-D serum (see p. 174), and a negative control such as AB (inert) serum. These controls must give the correct reaction patterns otherwise the results of that batch (plate) of tests are invalidated.

Enzyme techniques

External quality assessment schemes in the UK and elsewhere have consistently shown that enzyme techniques are capable of detecting low levels of many antibodies but are subject to false negative results and also to unwanted positive results, for example due to cold reactive antibodies and 'enzyme-only' panagglutinins. Microplate techniques are no exception to these problems and indeed their inherent sensitivity may exacerbate them. Low cell concentrations (less than 1%) of enzyme treated cells can be used in microplates to detect extremely low levels of antibody but are not suitable for routine antibody screening because of the greatly increased incidence of unwanted positive reactions. Sera which have a tendency to rouleaux formation will often give non-specific strongly positive reactions, or reaction patterns which are difficult to interpret. However prewarming sera and cells to 37°C will alleviate the problems caused by cold-reactive antibodies, and sera containing enzyme active panagglutinins can be diluted 1 + 1 with PBS and retested. This will usually allow any underlying alloantibodies to be detected.

The choice of bromelain or papain is subjective and laboratories may wish to continue to use their existing preparation. Preparation and QA of enzyme solutions are summarized in Appendix 3.

Two recommended enzyme techniques are listed below. The V-well technique is very sensitive but may be subject to more interference with enzyme-only panagglutinins than the U-well technique. Although reactions in the U-well technique can be interpreted on an automated plate reader, weak reactions will not be adequately determined.

Antiglobulin techniques

There are several important points to be considered when undertaking antiglobulin testing in microplates.

1 A wide range of cell concentrations can be used but a concentration of 3% is recommended because at this level problems of dilution and standardization of the antiglobulin reagent (see Appendix 6) are minimized and because the time taken for negative reactions to stream is reduced to an acceptable level.

2 Low or normal ionic strength solution (LISS or NISS) techniques can be used. LISS confers the same advantage in microplates as in tubes regarding time of incubation and has the additional advantage of requiring only 30–35 μl of serum per test, which will increase the efficiency of the washing phase (see below).

3 Resuspension techniques are not recommended for antiglobulin testing because of their lack of sensitivity. Streaming (trailing) techniques can be performed in U- or V-wells. A recommended V-well method is given on p. 180; those wishing to use a U-well method should note that centrifugation conditions may need to be adjusted.

4 Fully automated cell washers are now becoming available but their efficacy in liquid phase tests has yet to be established. Washing antiglobulin tests must therefore be done manually, although devices are available which can dispense wash fluid and aspirate supernatant quickly. There may be little or no time saved in antiglobulin testing in microplates compared with tube techniques for small blood banks. It is important during washing to remove as much supernatant as possible but without losing red cells and this is best achieved with a single flick action of the wrist (appropriate health and safety precautions should be taken). Five washes should be considered the minimum number acceptable for adequate removal of serum from all tests. Washing efficiency should be monitored regularly (see p. 181). Until efficient automated microplate washers become available, it is recommended that AHG control cells are used to confirm negative reactions. However these can only detect gross errors and should not be considered a substitute for a programme of regular monitoring.

5 The use of BSA and Tween 20 in the wash solution is a recommended measure for prevention of red cell monolayering (see p. 173) but albumin coating or pre-rinsing of microplates should not be necessary in the techniques described below.

6 A marked prozone may be encountered at incubation times greater than 2 minutes of AHG reagent with sensitized cells. It is therefore recommended that after addition of AHG reagent, tests are mixed and centrifuged immediately.

Layout

The layout of sera and cells in the microplate must be described in a laboratory Standard Operating Procedure (SOP) (see also p. 181).

Recommended enzyme technique for V-wells

1 Prepare a 3% suspension of enzyme-treated reagent red cells in a suitable diluent (see p. 173 and Appendix 4).

2 Add one drop (see p. 167) of test serum to the appropriate wells of a V-well microplate.

3 *Controls.* Add one drop of a weak anti-D control (see p. 174) and one drop of AB serum to the appropriate wells.

4 Add one drop of the 3% suspensions of enzyme treated reagent cells to the appropriate wells.

5 Agitate the plate to mix the reactants, preferably with a microplate shaker, taking care to ensure that no contamination occurs between wells.

6 Leave the plate at 37°C for 20–30 minutes and centrifuge at 150 g for 40 seconds (or suitable alternative rcf and time).

7 Check all tests for the presence of haemolysis if EDTA has not been added to the reagent cell diluent.

8 Place the microplate at an angle of about 70° to the horizontal and allow negative reactions to stream (trail). The exact length of time required for streaming will depend on a number of variables, for example centrifugation rcf, cell concentration and serum viscosity. The positive and negative controls must show correct reaction patterns.

9 Typical reaction patterns are shown in Figure 15.2.

Recommended enzyme technique for U-wells

1 Follow steps 1–5 above using a U-well microplate.

2 Leave the plate at 37°C for 20–30 minutes and centrifuge at 50 g for 4 minutes (or suitable alternative rcf and time).

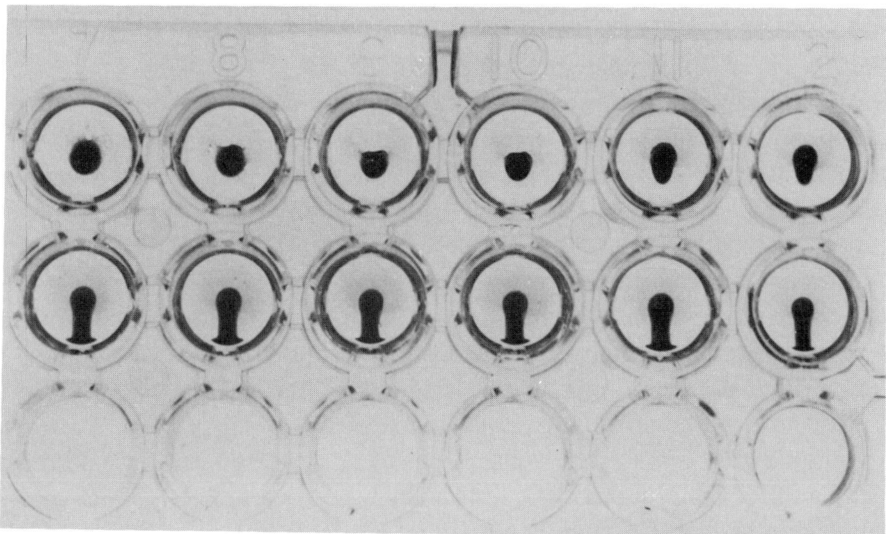

Fig. 15.2 Reaction patterns in a V-well streaming technique. Top row, left to right: four strongly positive reactions followed by two weakly positive reactions. Second row: negative reactions.

3 Check all tests for the presence of haemolysis if EDTA has not been added to the reagent cell diluent.
4 Resuspend the red cells using a microplate shaker as described on p. 175.
5 Typical reaction patterns are shown in Figure 15.1. The use of a magnifying mirror allows reactions to be read from underneath and this is particularly helpful in determining weak reactions.

Recommended indirect antiglobulin technique for V-wells

1 Prepare a 3% suspension of reagent red cells in a suitable diluent i.e. LISS or NISS (see pp. 173 & 177).
2 Add one drop (see p. 167) of test serum for LISS techniques, or two drops for NISS techniques, to the appropriate wells of a V-well microplate.
3 *Controls.* Add one drop of a weak anti-D control (see p. 174) and one drop of AB serum to the appropriate wells.
4 Add one drop of the 3% suspensions of reagent cells to the appropriate wells.
5 Agitate the plate to mix the reactants, preferably with a microplate shaker, taking care to ensure that no contamination occurs between wells.
6 Leave the plate at 37°C for 20–60 minutes (LISS techniques) or 45–60 minutes (NISS techniques).
7 Check all tests for the presence of haemolysis if EDTA has not been added to the reagent cell diluent.
8 Wash the tests five times by the following method.

(a) Add approximately 150 µl wash fluid (PBS containing 0.1% BSA and 0.02% Tween 20) so that each well is almost full.

(b) Centrifuge the plate so that red cells are sedimented; this can be achieved rapidly by switching off the centrifuge as soon as 800 g is reached.

(c) Decant the supernatant by a flick action or by using an aspirating device.

(d) Resuspend cell buttons completely during washing by using a microplate shaker and/or the force of the wash fluid jet.

9 After decanting the final wash, add two drops of AHG reagent to each well, and agitate the plate carefully but thoroughly mix the reactants.
10 Centrifuge the plate immediately at 150 g for 40 seconds.
11 Read reaction patterns as described above (1–9).
12 Add one drop of 3% AHG control cells to all negative reactions and repeat steps 10 and 11. Confirm that these tests are now positive; any tests which remain negative must be repeated. A suitable method for the preparation of AHG control cells is given in Chapter 14.

Batching of tests

Batching of tests is particularly useful when blood grouping in microplates as the 96-well format allows large numbers of tests to be conveniently set up and read. Batching also allows economy in the use of controls, as each batch of tests should contain one set of relevant controls. The appropriate controls for each technique are described in the relevant sections. For this purpose a batch of tests is defined as one or more microplates which:

1 have the same layout of antiserum and reagent red cells in the rows or columns of the microplate(s);

2 have the same batches of reagent red cells and batch/lot numbers of antisera throughout;

3 are from the same manufacturer with the same product number;

4 have all test sera and antisera dispensed from the same size pipette, and similarly for test cells and reagent cells;

5 have all test cells suspended in the same diluent (from the same batch);

6 are tested by the same person(s);

7 are performed in one run at one time;

8 have all antiglobulin tests washed using the same batch of saline or wash fluid.

Quality assurance

Quality assurance (QA) should consist of the following factors.

1 Reagent evaluation, if the reagents are not standardized for microplate use (see Appendix 6).

2 Pre-acceptance or batch testing prior to routine use (see Appendix 7).

3 Validation of any new procedure in the laboratory by comparison with established tube techniques (see Appendix 8).

4 Daily or batch controls (see pp. 174 & 177).

5 Routine checking of the washing efficiency in antiglobulin testing (at least twice a week) using at least one plate of replicate tests with 1+/2+ sensitized cells (Chapter 14).

These should all be performed following the laboratory's written Standard Operating Procedures (SOPs) (Chapter 19), the results properly recorded and these records examined by a nominated QA officer or senior scientist. Corrective action should be taken as appropriate and recorded.

Details of dates of receipt, lot numbers, expiry dates and storage conditions should always be kept. If reagents are diluted or used in a way not recommended by the manufacturer then product liability no longer rests with the manufacturer but with the user, and hence it is important to keep accurate records of standardization procedures, dilution factor and details of the diluent. These records must be signed and dated.

Documentation is covered in Chapters 12 and 13.

Appendix 1: Phosphate buffered saline (PBS)

Saline should be buffered to pH 6.8–7.2 at 20°C and the buffering capacity should be sufficient to maintain the pH during the shelf-life of the saline. PBS suitable for serological use is available from several commercial sources.

Appendix 2: EDTA solution for diluents

Stock solution: prepare a 0.1 mol/l solution of EDTA (dipotassium salt) in distilled water. Adjust the pH to 7.0 with 5 mol/l NaOH.

Working solution: mix one volume of stock solution with nine volumes of PBS or LISS. Check the pH and adjust to 7.0 if necessary.

Appendix 3: Enzyme solutions

Bromelain has historically been the enzyme of choice in blood grouping in microplates, but bromelain or papain is usually used for antibody screening. Suggested methods of preparation are given below (enzyme techniques and reference standards are currently being investigated by a working party set up by the International Society of Blood Transfusion and the International Committee for Standardization in Haematology). Note that enzyme powders may be allergenic and irritants. A face mask should therefore be worn when handling these materials.

1 BROMELAIN PREPARATION

A 0.1% (w/v) bromelain extract in saline will normally give satisfactory results. Bromelain powder may be obtained from Hughes and Hughes Ltd (Romford, Essex) or Sigma Chemical Co. Ltd. (Poole, Dorset).

Stock solution. Add 5 ml PBS to 1 g of bromelain powder and mix to a paste with an applicator stick. Add 85 ml PBS and 10 ml of EDTA stock solution (see Appendix 2) and mix well for 5 minutes. Centrifuge the suspension to precipitate insoluble material and save the supernatant. Measure the pH of this stock solution which should not vary from batch to batch. The enzyme activity of the stock solution can be assayed biochemically using a suitable method which is useful in eliminating variation between new and current batches of bromelain. The stock solution should be stored at − 30°C or below unless used within 24 hours.

Working solution. Dilute the stock solution 1 + 9 with PBS, or to a predetermined level of enzyme activity if a biochemical assay has been used. Each batch of working strength solution should be tested in the appropriate technique with a known weak anti-D serum (see p. 174) which should give a macroscopic positive reaction with D pos (preferably R_1r) cells and an inert AB serum should give a negative reaction. This testing should be performed using the two-stage (Appendix 4) or one-stage (Appendix 5) techniques by which the reagent will be used. Working strength solution should be given a shelf-life of 24 hours.

2 PAPAIN PREPARATION

A 0.1% (w/v) papain extract in saline will normally give satisfactory results. Papain powder may be obtained from Sigma Chemical Co. Ltd. (Poole, Dorset).

0.5 mol/l cysteine. Dissolve 0.88 g L-cysteine hydrochloride in 10 ml distilled water.

pH 5.4 saline. Mix 3.5 ml of 0.1 mol/l Na_2HPO_4, 96.5 ml of 0.1 mol/l KH_2PO_4 and 900 ml of 0.15mol/l NaC1. Check and adjust the pH to 5.4 with 0.1 mol/l Na_2HPO_4 or 0.1 mol/l KH_2PO_4.

Papain stock solution. Add 2 g papain powder to 100 ml of pH 5.4 saline and shake well for 15 minutes. Centrifuge and/or filter to remove the debris. Add 10 ml of 0.5 mol/l cysteine, and make up to 200 ml with pH 5.4 saline. Incubate at 37°C for 30 minutes. The enzyme activity of the stock solution can be assayed biochemically to eliminate batch to batch variation. The stock solution should be stored at – 30°C or below unless used within 24 hours.

Papain working solution. Dilute the stock solution 1 + 9 with PBS, or to a predetermined level of enzyme activity if a biochemical assay has been used. Quality assurance and shelf-life of the solution is as described for bromelain solution (see Appendix 3).

Appendix 4: Two stage enzyme treatment of reagent cells

See pp. 172, 173 and 177 for the application of two-stage enzyme techniques in reverse ABO grouping and antibody screening. The time and temperature conditions given for enzyme treatment below are likely to give good results in antibody screening. QA must demonstrate the efficacy of enzyme treatment and the appropriate conditions must be clearly documented in a laboratory SOP. Bromelain and papain treated cells should be stored at 4°C when not in use, up to a maximum of 24 hours.

Mix two volumes of working strength solution (see Appendix 3) with one volume of washed, packed cells and incubate at 37°C for 15 minutes. Wash twice in PBS and resuspend to 3% in EDTA/PBS (see Appendix 2) or in PBS.

Appendix 5: One-stage bromelain technique for blood grouping

See p. 171 for the application of one-stage enzyme techniques in ABO and D grouping of red cells.

Packed cells are suspended in the working strength bromelain solution (Appendix 3) to give a 3% suspension and this is used directly (without washing) as described on p. 175. If the red cell suspension is to be kept for more than 60 minutes, however, the cells should be washed twice in PBS and stored at 4°C for use up to 24 hours.

Appendix 6: Evaluation and standardization of reagents for microplate use

The following sections give recommended minimum requirements when using reagents not standardized for the methods described on pp. 175 and 180.

1 ABO GROUPING REAGENTS

1 Make serial (doubling) dilutions of the reagent in an appropriate diluent (see pp. 170 and 171).
2 Test these dilutions using the method given on p. 175 with at least the following numbers of phenotype examples. ABO antigens are less developed in the red cells of newborn infants than in adults and therefore cord cells from group A or AB infants and from B or AB infants may be used instead of A_2B and A_1B cells, respectively, for testing anti-A and anti-B. However, the strength of ABO antigens in cord samples is highly variable, and it is recommended that 5 examples should be tested. Note that the strength of the A antigen in A_x red cells is also highly variable between different examples. Grade each reaction on a scale from 0 (negative) to 4 (complete agglutination).

Anti-A 1 A_1, 1 A_2, 3 A_2B, 1 O
Anti-B 2 B, 3 A_1B, 1 O
Anti-A,B 1 A_1, 2 A_2, 1 A_x, 2 B, 1 O

3 Select a dilution that if it were further diluted 1 + 3 would give at least the following strength reactions with the following reactors:

Anti-A 4+ with A_1 and A_2 cells, 3+ with A_2B cells
Anti-B 4+ with A_1B and B cells
Anti-A,B 4+ with A_1, A_2 and B cells, 2+ with A_x cells

2 Rh D GROUPING REAGENTS

1 Make serial (doubling) dilutions of the anti-D reagent in an appropriate diluent (see pp. 170 and 171).
2 Test these dilutions using the method given on p. 175 with at least 3 examples of the R_1r phenotype or 10 random D positive (not D^u) samples. Grade each reaction on a scale from 0 (negative) to 4 (complete agglutination).
3 Select a dilution that gives 4+ reactions with all samples, 4+ reactions if further diluted 1 + 1 and at least a 1+ reaction with the weakest reactor if diluted 1 + 7.

3 ANTIGLOBULIN (AHG) REAGENTS

Voak *et al.*, 1986; Engelfriet *et al.*, 1987; and ISBT/ICSH, 1987 give useful information about the important characteristics of antiglobulin reagents.

1 Make serial dilutions of the AHG reagent in 1% BSA in PBS, up to a maximum dilution of 1 : 16. Caution: all manipulations using AHG reagent and washed cells must be performed using clean pipettes and glassware.

2 Perform three 'chequerboard' titrations as follows.

(a) Select three non-saline reactive sera (anti-D, anti-Kell and anti-Fy^a) which give titres of 8–16 when tested using an appropriate spin tube technique (LISS or NISS) with heterozygous cells. Make serial (doubling) dilutions of the sera in 1% BSA in PBS from neat to 1 : 128.

(b) Prepare in LISS or NISS 10 ml of 3% red cells of the appropriate phenotype for each of the sera to be tested (e.g. R_1r, K + k + and Fy(a+b+)).

(c) Add one drop (two drops for NISS techniques) of undiluted anti-D to five wells (columns 1 to 5) of row A of a V-well microplate. Add one drop (two drops for NISS) of anti-D diluted 1 : 2 to five wells of row B of this plate. Repeat for each anti-D dilution up to 1 : 128 using rows C to H.

(d) Continue the antiglobulin test as on p. 180 (4 to 8).

(e) Decant the final wash. Add two drops of undiluted AHG to the eight test wells in row A. Add two drops of AHG diluted 1 : 2 to the eight test wells in column 2. Repeat for each AHG dilution up to 1 : 16 using columns 3 to 5.

(f) Agitate the plate carefully to mix the reactants thoroughly and continue as on p. 180 (10 to 12). Typical results for a chequerboard titration are shown in Table 15.1.

(g) Repeat steps (c)–(f) above for the anti-Kell and anti-Fy^a.

3 (a) Prepare one batch of complement coated cells, using for example a non-agglutinating complement-binding anti-Le^a or anti-Le^b serum which has been freshly obtained.

Alternatively, iC3b and C3d coated cells can be reliably produced *in vitro* using a low ionic strength sucrose method (Voak *et al.*, 1986; Engelfriet *et al.*, 1987).

(b) Prepare three batches of cells which are direct antiglobulin test negative.

(c) Prepare one batch of bromelain or papain treated cells (direct antiglobulin test negative before enzyme treatment). See Appendix 4 for suggested methods of enzyme treatment.

(d) Cells prepared in steps (a) to (c) above should be washed thoroughly in PBS (remember that at least six washes may be necessary for large volumes of packed cells), resuspended to 3% in PBS and their reactivity or non-reactivity with AHG reagent

Table A1 Chequerboard titration of an anti-D serum tested with anti-human globulin reagent in a microplate technique.

Anti-D dilution	AHG dilution Neat	1 : 2	1 : 4	1 : 8	1 : 16
Neat	4 + *	4 +	4 +	4 +	4 +
1 : 2	4 +	4 +	4 +	4 +	4 +
1 : 4	2 +	3 +	3 +	3 +	3 +
1 : 8	1 +	2 +	2 +	3 +	2 +
1 : 16	0	0	0	0	0

* Grade of reaction on a scale 0 (negative) to 4 + (complete).

confirmed by testing in a tube direct antiglobulin test. Cells prepared in step (a) should be shown to be negative with an anti-IgG reagent.

(e) Test each dilution of AHG reagent against each 3% cell suspension prepared in steps 3(a) to (3c) above as described on p. 180 (9 to 12). Each cell suspension should also be tested with diluent (1% BSA in PBS) only.

4 Select the strongest AHG reagent dilution which gives optimal reactivity with weakly sensitized cells in the chequerboard titrations. This dilution should be positive with cells prepared in step 3 (a) and negative with cells prepared in steps 3 (b)–(c).

4 STORAGE OF DILUTED REAGENTS

If reagents for ABO, D or antiglobulin testing are to be diluted it is recommended that this is done on a daily basis. Diluents such as PBS or 1% BSA in PBS should also be made daily. Working strength reagents should be stored at 4°C when not in use; stock (undiluted) reagents should be stored according to the manufacturers' instructions, with due reference to the expiry date. The life of working strength reagents may be prolonged by the addition of sodium azide to a final concentration of 1 g/l but if this is done then it should be shown and documented that there is no loss of activity during the storage period.

Appendix 7: Pre-acceptance testing

Each batch of all reagents, including those which have been restandardized and diluted, should be examined prior to general use. Reagents should not be used if a precipitate, a gel, particles or turbidity is present. Routine microplate techniques described in the laboratory SOPs should be used to monitor potency and specificity as described below.

ABO AND D GROUPING REAGENTS

ABO reagents: test at least one example of each of A_1, A_2, A_1B, A_2B, B and O.
Anti-D reagents: test at least one example of each of A_1rr, Brr, Orr, R_1r, r″r and r′r.

POLYSPECIFIC ANTI-HUMAN GLOBULIN REAGENTS

Compare the performance of the new reagent with the reagent currently in use, using a selection of weak (preferably undiluted) warm reacting IgG antibodies reactive in the indirect anti-globulin technique.

Test the reagent for freedom from false positive reactions by 'cross-matching' 10 fresh group compatible sera against red cells from at least 10 donor pack integral segment lines stored 28 to 35 days at 4°C (i.e. a minimum of 10 tests).

BOVINE SERUM ALBUMIN (BSA) FOR USE AS A DILUENT OR DILUENT CONTROL

Dilute previously standardized ABO and D grouping and antiglobulin reagents to concentrations established in Appendix 6. Use a diluent containing the previously used batch of BSA and test in parallel with a diluent containing the new batch of BSA using the protocols for pre-acceptance testing described above. Positive reactions obtained with the reagents suspended in both diluents should be comparably avid. Negative reactions should be resuspended (ABO and D grouping reagents) or should stream (antiglobulin reagents) without difficulty using both diluents.

Appendix 8: Validation of a liquid-phase microplate technique

Any new technique should be tested in parallel with existing techniques before being introduced into routine laboratory use. The following sections give an additional formal assurance of the efficacy of microplate techniques by *validation* with standard tube methods.

1 ABO AND D GROUPING

1 Proceed as in Appendix 6, section 1, steps 1–2, and Appendix 6, section 2, steps 1–2. In addition test these dilutions with the same cells but using the (tube) technique(s) recommended by the manufacturer(s) of the antisera.

2 The microplate method should give results, using antisera at the intended dilutions, which are comparable with the results obtained in the tube technique(s) using undiluted antisera. Titres obtained using the various cells give an indication of the relative robustness of tube and microplate techniques.

2 ENZYME ANTIBODY SCREENING TECHNIQUE

1 Select at least three sera (e.g. anti-D, -c and -E) which give titres of 8–16 when tested using an appropriate tube technique with enzyme treated cells. Make serial (doubling) dilutions of the sera in 1% BSA in PBS. Test these dilutions using the selected microplate method (see pp. 178 and 179 and Appendix 4 for recommended methods) and using the tube method with enzyme treated cells of the appropriate phenotype.

2 Select 5–10 sera of known blood group specificity which are known to be weakly reactive using the enzyme tube method. In addition select 5–10 sera which are known to be non-reactive using the enzyme tube method. Test all sera using the microplate method and using the tube method with enzyme treated cells of the appropriate phenotype (blood group specific sera should be tested with cells containing and lacking the appropriate antigens).

3 The microplate method should give results which are comparable with the results obtained in the tube method. The comparative titrations give an indication of the relative sensitivity of the methods. If there is a consistently high level of unwanted positive results then the procedure should be reviewed.

3 ANTIGLOBULIN ANTIBODY SCREENING TECHNIQUE

1 Proceed as in Appendix 6, section 3, steps 1, 2, 3(a) and 3 (d)–(e). In addition perform these tests using an appropriate LISS or NISS spin tube technique.

2 Select 5–10 sera of known blood group specificity which are known to be weakly reactive using the antiglobulin spin tube method. In addition select 5–10 sera which are known to be non-reactive using this method. Test all sera using the microplate method and using the spin tube method with cells of the appropriate phenotype (blood group specific sera should be tested with cells containing and lacking the appropriate antigens).

3 The microplate method should generally give results which are at least as good as or better than the results obtained in the tube method. The titrations give an indication of the relative sensitivity of the methods and also demonstrate whether prozone is encountered using IgG sensitized cells in the microplate method. There should not be any evidence of monolayering or unwanted positive results. (Freedom from false positives is further assessed in pre-acceptance testing which is dealt with in Appendix 7.)

References

Bowley A.R., Gordon I. & Ross D.W. (1984) Computer controlled automated reading of blood groups using microplates. *Medical Laboratory Sciences* **41**, 19–28.

Crawford M.N., Gottman F.E. & Gottman C.A. (1970) Microplate system for routine use in blood bank laboratories. *Transfusion* **10**, 258–263.

Doughty R.W. (1989) Product liability in the medical laboratory, *Medical Laboratory Sciences* **46**, 68–71.

Engelfriet C.P., Overbeeke M.A.M. & Voak D. (1987) The antiglobulin test (Coombs test) and the red cell. In Cash J.D. (ed.) *Progress in Transfusion Medicine Vol. 2*, pp. 74–98. Churchill Livingstone, Edinburgh.

ISBT/ICSH Working Party (1987) International reference polyspecific anti-globulin reagents. *Vox Sanguinis* **53**, 241–247.

Parker J.L., Marcoux D.A., Hafleigh E.B. & Grumet F.C. (1978) Modified microtiter tray method for blood typing. *Transfusion* **18**, 417–422.

Sever J.L. (1962) Application of a microtechnique to viral serological investigations. *Journal of Immunology* **88**, 320–329.

Severns M.L., Schoeppner S.L., Cozart M.J., Friedman L.I. & Schanfield M.S. (1984) Automated determination of ABO/Rh in microplates. *Vox Sanguinis* **47**, 293–303.

Voak D., Downie D.M., Moore B.P.L. & Engelfriet C.P. (1986) Anti-human globulin reagent specification: the European and ISBT/ICSH view. *Biotest Bulletin* **3**, 7–22.

Warlow A. & Tills D. (1978) Micromethods in blood group serology. *Vox Sanguinis* **35**, 354–356.

Wegmann T.G. & Smithies O. (1966) A simple hemagglutination system requiring small amounts of red cells and antibodies. *Transfusion* **6**, 67–73.

Wegmann T.G. & Smithies O. (1968) Improvement of the microtiter hemagglutination method. *Transfusion* **8**, 47.

16 Implementation of a Maximum Surgical Blood Order Schedule

Prepared by the
Blood Transfusion Task Force

Introduction

Blood transfusion laboratories have experienced gradually increasing workloads without any corresponding increase in trained staff; this has become more acute during the past 5 years. New procedures to reduce unnecessary workload and stress are vital to improve the efficiency of the service. A reappraisal and rationalization of compatibility procedures (see Chapter 14) and the introduction of maximum surgical blood order schedules are important developments in this respect (Friedman *et al.*, 1976; Dodsworth & Dudlety, 1985; Napier *et al.*, 1985; Perrault & Barr, 1986).

The Maximum Surgical Blood Order Schedule (MSBOS) is a table of elective surgical procedures which lists the number of units of blood routinely cross-matched for them pre-operatively.

The schedule is based on a retrospective analysis of actual blood usage associated with the individual surgical procedure. It aims to correlate as closely as possible the amount of blood cross-matched (C) to the amount of blood transfused (T). The C : T ratio can be used to monitor the efficiency of the scheme.

The introduction of an MSBOS has the following advantages.

1 A reduction in cross-matching workload of the blood transfusion laboratory (in some cases in excess of 25%) which allows more time to respond to emergency requests, and also to investigate complex serological problems.

2 A reduction in the level of stress.

3 More efficient use of blood stocks and a reduction in wastage due to out-dating.

An important factor in the establishment of an MSBOS is the identification of those procedures that can be accommodated by the group, antibody screen and save procedure.

Surgical procedures will normally fall into two categories.

1 Those catered for by group and antibody screen only ('G & S'). If the antibody screen is negative, no blood is cross-matched and the serum is saved.

2 Those for which blood is cross-matched according to the schedule.

The system *allows for flexibility*. If patients in the 'G & S' category have a positive antibody screen, antigen negative cross-matched blood must be made available. If the clinical circumstances indicate that extra blood may be required for a particular patient, extra units may be cross-matched. However, exceeding the 'tariff' must be monitored to prevent abuse of the system.

Serological techniques

A blood sample from all surgical patients must have a full ABO and Rh D group and antibody screen, as described in Chapter 14.

For patients in the 'G & S' category, if the serum is to be saved for cross-matching, it should be separated and frozen at −20°C or below within 24 hours of collection, be accurately labelled and readily accessible. Under normal circumstances an upper storage limit of 2 weeks is advisable.

Antibodies are more likely to appear in antenatal patients and those transfused during the preceding 3 months. For this reason it is recommended that a fresh sample is obtained for compatibility testing if more than 3 days have elapsed since the original sample was collected.

If blood is required urgently for any surgical patient, blood of the same ABO and Rh D group can be given after cross-matching by the appropriate rapid procedures depending on the time available (see Chapter 14).

Constructing the tariff

A draft schedule of expected blood usage (or 'tariff') for each surgical procedure is produced by analysing the hospital blood usage data. The use of computers greatly facilitates this. It is necessary to analyse data retrospectively for all surgical cross-match requests over at least a 6-month period. It is important to collect a sufficient number of each procedure to give a meaningful assessment, and to exclude the exceptional massive transfusion cases that might bias the result. The data should be analysed for each procedure to indicate the number of units cross-matched, the number of units transfused, the percentage used, the C : T ratio and the average number of units transfused for each procedure (see Table 16.1).

The ideal value for the C : T ratio is 1 : 1. The higher the value the more blood that is being cross-matched unnecessarily. A realistic objective for surgical procedures is a C : T ratio of between 3 : 1 and 2 : 1, which corresponds to a blood usage of between approximately 30 and 50%.

Table 16.1 Example of analysis of transfusion data for some selected operative procedures

Operation	No. of operations	No. of units cross-matched	No. of units transfused	% Units transfused	C:T ratio
*TURP	134	292	30	10.2	9.7:1
Abdominal hysterectomy	93	216	39	18.0	5.5:1
Colectomy	47	188	87	46.2	2.1:1

* TURP = trans-urethral resection of prostate

In constructing the draft schedule, procedures that have a blood usage of less than 30% are allocated to the 'G & S' category. Other procedures are allotted a 'tariff' based on the average number of units transfused.

In drawing up the 'tariff' allowance must be made for local factors that would affect the speed of provision of compatible blood, such as the distance of operating theatres from the blood transfusion laboratory and portering (transport) arrangements. Haematologists responsible for the supply of blood to nursing homes and private hospitals approved for abortion by the Secretary of State should consult the guidelines prepared by the Department of Health (Appendix 1).

An example of a typical MSBOS is given in Appendix 2. It should be emphasized that local circumstances and clinical practice may occasionally appear to bias the tariff in favour of some procedures.

Implementation

It is essential from the start to obtain the confidence of the surgical and anaesthetic teams. Initial contact should be made to explain the proposal to introduce an MSBOS and to let them know that data on surgical procedures is being collected and analysed. Once the draft schedule has been drawn up it should be circulated to the surgeons and anaesthetists for discussion. The consultant haematologist should then meet with each surgical team and describe the MSBOS, explain the local arrangements for providing compatible blood quickly in an emergency and negotiate an agreed 'tariff' for their particular specialty for incorporation in the proposed schedule. It should also be explained that the system allows for flexibility as previously described.

The accepted schedule should be distributed to all relevant staff, preferably in a pocket-sized format. Instruction in the use of MSBOS should be part of the induction course for junior medical staff.

Monitoring is required to detect medical staff who disregard the system or who distrust the ability of the laboratory to provide blood in an emergency. Education of recurrent 'offenders' is better than harassment to promote compliance.

Revision

The schedule should be reviewed regularly and adjustments made as necessary for 'fine tuning'. This is much easier to achieve if the laboratory is computerized.

Operation

Confidence in the operation of MSBOS and compliance by users depends on the laboratory being able to provide compatible blood whenever it is required, including urgent requests. This is dependent on the following five factors.

1 Pre-operative blood samples must be obtained from all patients in the 'G & S' and cross-matching categories. The laboratory will normally set its own time limits for the receipt of blood for grouping and antibody screening before operation. If an irregular antibody is detected, this may delay the provision of compatible blood and the consultant must be informed.

2 Serum saved for cross-matching must be accurately labelled and readily accessible.

3 Procedures must be clearly defined to enable blood transfusion staff to provide compatible blood safely should an emergency occur during a 'G & S' operation.

4 Communication between the operating theatre and the blood transfusion laboratory must be clearly defined. An urgent need for blood during an operation must be promptly reported to the laboratory by the anaesthetist, or his/her deputy. The request must be received by a responsible person in the blood transfusion laboratory (usually a technologist/MLSO) and acted upon immediately. Adequate details to identify the patient are essential and the degree of urgency must be clearly indicated so that the most appropriate compatibility tests can be carried out in the time available.

5 Portering of blood between the laboratory and the operating theatre must have an established priority.

Appendix 1

Revised guidelines for routine blood testing and emergency blood cover for nursing homes and private hospitals approved for abortion by the Secretary of State

PRE-OPERATIVE ROUTINE BLOOD TESTING FOR ABORTION PATIENTS

1 *All patients* to be tested and the results to be available at the nursing home or hospital before operation:

(a) haemoglobin

(b) blood group (A, B, O and Rhesus (D))
(c) screen for atypical *red cell antibodies.*

2 *All patients.* The blood group to be performed and a sample of serum held in advance by the hospital blood bank or private laboratory which can provide a 24-hour service for cross-matching if required.

Note. Facilities should be available to enable screening for such conditions as sickle-cell disorders to be performed where indicated.

BLOOD SUPPLIES AND OTHER IV FLUIDS REQUIRED IN AN EMERGENCY

1 Available immediately at the nursing home or hospital:
(a) Plasma protein fraction (minimum 2 units of 500 ml) or albumin 4/5% (minimum 2 units of 500 ml)
(b) Plasma protein substitute (minimum 4 litres)
(c) Crystalloid IV solutions (including dextrose saline and electrolyte solutions)

2 Available immediately or within 15 minutes of requirement:
(a) Either two units of O Rhesus-negative blood to be available for use *within 15 minutes* (either held at the nursing home or hospital or 'ear-marked' for them and held in an adjacent hospital blood bank or private laboratory); or if two units of O Rhesus-negative blood cannot be guaranteed within 15 minutes, two units of blood to be cross-matched in advance, *before the operation* is performed.
(b) *For all cases,* found on screening to have atypical *red cell antibodies,* two units of blood to be cross-matched in advance *before the operation* is performed.

3 Available if the emergency continues:
(a) Supplies of cross-matched blood should be 'rapidly obtainable' in an emergency (not more than 60 minutes). This time should take into account geographical distance and travelling conditions at the busiest times of the day.
(b) As described above *in all cases* serum should be held in advance at the hospital blood bank or private laboratory for cross-matching if required.

4 If the emergency blood supplies available at the home or private hospital have been used up the operation list must be suspended until they have been replaced.

5 The nursing homes or private hospitals should have suitable blood refrigerators solely reserved for blood storage. The supplies of blood should be supervised by a haematologist and made available for recycling if possible.

August 1989
Department of Health and Social Security
Alexander Fleming House
Elephant and Castle, London SE1 6BY
(Tel: 071-407 5522 ext. 7292/6973)

Appendix 2

A Maximum Surgical Blood Order Schedule prepared to meet the needs of a large teaching hospital

SURGICAL BLOOD ORDERING TARIFF

General surgery

Cholecystectomy and exploration of common duct	G & S
Splenectomy	G & S
Laparotomy—planned exploration	G & S
Liver biopsy	G & S
Vagotomy +/− drainage	G & S
Gastrostomy, ileostomy, colostomy	G & S
Oesophageal dilation	G & S
Oesophagectomy	5
Hiatus hernia	2
Partial gastrectomy	G & S
Oesophagogastrectomy	4
Hepatectomy	4
Mastectomy (simple)	G & S
Endocrine	
Thyroidectomy—partial/total	G & S
Parathyroidectomy	G & S
Adrenalectomy	3
Pancreatectomy—partial/Whipple	4
Transplantation	
Renal	2
Graft nephrectomy	2
Donor nephrectomy	G & S
Marrow harvest	2

Colo-rectal surgery

Rectum—pouch; resection/excision etc.	2
Intra-abdominal—colectomy etc.	2
Rectopexy	G & S

Vascular surgery

Amputation of leg	G & S
Sympathectomy	G & S
Femoral endarterectomy	G & S
Carotid endarterectomy	G & S
Femoro-popliteal bypass	2
Axillo-femoral bypass	2
Aorto-femoral bypass	4

Bifemoral bypass	6
Aorto-iliac bypass	4
Aorto-iliac endartectomy	4
Infra-renal aortic aneurysm	6
Thoracic or thoraco-abdominal aneurysm	10
Ruptured aneurysms	10

Cardio-thoracic surgery

Angloplasty	G & S
Open heart operations—CAVBG, MVR, AVR, (re-do*)	4 (8*)
Bronchoscopy	G & S
Open pleural/lung biopsy	G & S
Lobectomy/pneumonectomy	2
Sternal refashioning	G & S

Neurosurgery

Head injury, extradural haematoma	2
Craniotomy, craniectomy	G & S
Meningioma	4
Vascular surgery (aneurysms, A–V malformations)	3
Shunt procedures	G & S
Cranioplasty	G & S
Trans-sphenoidal hypophysectomy	G & S
Vascular transformations, posterior fossa exploration	2
Disc surgery	G & S
Laminectomy	G & S
Spinal decompression for tumours	2
Peripheral nerve surgery	G & S

Orthopaedics

Removal hip pin or femoral nail	G & S
Osteotomy/bone biopsy (except upper femur *)	G & S (2*)
Removal cervical rib	G & S
Bone graft from iliac crest—1 side (both sides *)	G & S (2*)
Nailing fractured neck of femur	G & S
Spinal fusion	2
Laminectomy	G & S
Internal fixation of femur	2
Internal fixation—tibia or ankle	G & S
Arthroplasty—total knee or shoulder	2
—total hip	2
—total elbow	2
Changing hip prosthesis	4
Dynamic hip screw	G & S

Urology

Cystectomy	6
Cystectomy and urethrectomy	8
Nephrectomy	2
Nephrectomy and expioration of vena cava	6
Open nephrolithotomy	2
Open prostatectomy (RPP)	2
TURP	G & S
TUR bladder tumour (large tumour)	G & S
Percutaneous nephrolithotomy	G & S
Ureterolithotomy	G & S
Cystotomy	G & S
Ureterolithotomy and cystotomy	G & S
Reimplantation of ureter	G & S
Urethroplasty	2

Head and neck

Major H–N procedures—laryngectomy etc.	2
Major plastic reconstructions (see Plastic surgery)	
Other H–N procedures	G & S

Plastic surgery

Abdominoplasty	G & S
Mammoplasty	G & S
Head and neck reconstructions	2

Dental

Trauma and reconstructions	2

Obstetrics and gynaecology

LSCS	G & S
ERPC/D & C	G & S
Hydatidiform mole	2
Placenta praevia/retained placenta	2
APH/PPH	2 (variable)
Hysterectomy: abdominal or vaginal—simple	G & S
—extended	2
Werthelm's operation	4
Pelvic exenteration	6
Vulvectomy (radical)	4
Myomectomy	2
Oophorectomy (radical)	4
Termination of pregnancy	G & S

References

Dodsworth H. & Dudley H.A.F. (1985) Increased efficiency of transfusion practice in routine surgery using pre-operative antibody screening and selective ordering with an abbreviated cross-match. *British Journal of Surgery* **72**, 102–104.

Friedman B.A., Oberman H.A., Chadwick A.R. & Kingdon K.I. (1976) The maximum surgical blood order schedule and surgical blood use in the United States. *Transfusion* **16**, 380–387.

Napier J.A.F., Biffin A.H. & Lay D. (1985) Efficiency of use of blood for surgery in south and mid Wales. *British Medical Journal* **291**, 799–801.

Perrault R.A. & Barr R.A. (1986) Blood ordering strategies. In Cash J.D. (ed.) *Progress in Transfusion Medicine, 1*, pp. 95–107 Churchill Livingstone, Edinburgh.

17 Transfusion for Massive Blood Loss

Prepared by the
Blood Transfusion Task Force

These guidelines have been prepared in an attempt to summarize current opinions regarding the management of massive transfusions and also to identify those areas where unjustified therapy should be curtailed. In this regard it should be borne in mind that many of the currently established transfusion practices are based more on benefits that are hoped for than those that have been proven. These notes make no attempt to resolve the numerous highly contentious issues surrounding aspects of transfusion therapy in this situation.

Massive blood loss is a catastrophe which presents a serious threat to survival. This danger may create extreme tensions between those attempting to treat the haemorrhage, those supplying blood or blood components, and the staff providing laboratory services. Such circumstances can cause waste of scarce transfusion materials or, even worse, result in mistakes that can contribute to the death of the patient.

Definition of massive transfusion

This is somewhat arbitrary but is commonly accepted to entail transfusion of a volume equal to the patient's total blood volume in less than 24 hours. The management strategy is therefore focused towards patients who, for example, arrive in casualty exsanguinating, or towards surgical or obstetric patients presenting with overwhelming haemorrhage. It should be emphasized that, unless there are pre-existing abnormalities of haemostasis or plasma protein composition, the haematological problems to be discussed should not be expected for transfusion rates less than those mentioned above.

Aim of treatment

The blood transfusion strategy should be to maintain blood composition within limits that are safe with regard to haemostasis, blood oxygen-carrying capacity, oncotic pressure and plasma biochemistry.

Reprinted with permission from *Clinical and Laboratory Haematology*, 1988, **10**, 265–273.

High-risk patients

Massively transfused patients do not form a homogeneous group in which complications can be predicted. Conservative management protocols must therefore take account of the possibility that pre-existing high-risk factors may not have been accurately identified. It must be recognized, however, that these problems may accelerate the appearance of transfusion complications.

Prolonged hypotension and shock predispose to disseminated intravascular coagulation and adult respiratory distress syndrome. Delayed treatment of shock is probably the most important factor predisposing to problems during resuscitation.

Adult respiratory distress syndrome is believed to be more likely in patients with persistent congestive cardiac failure, sepsis, and those who are either undertransfused or overtransfused.

Extensive tissue damage, particularly involving head injuries, can also be associated with coagulation disturbances. Patients with severe head injuries may also be at risk of cerebral oedema if plasma oncotic pressure is allowed to fall excessively.

Patients with hepatic or renal failure may not only have abnormalities of haemostasis or plasma proteins but may also have impaired metabolic responses to the citrate, potassium or glucose infused with stored blood.

Problems of massive transfusion

Blood volume replacement

Many of the complications of massive transfusion are aggravated by either under- or over-transfusion. Judgement of the adequacy of transfusion is a skilled clinical matter, discussion of which is beyond the scope of this chapter. As a minimum, normal systolic pressures and pulse rate, a urine output of at least 30 ml/hour and haematocrit values of 0.32 are indicative of acceptable blood transfusion replacement.

Thrombocytopenia

Blood which has been stored for more than a few days is devoid of functioning platelets; dilutional thrombocytopenia is therefore to be anticipated during massive blood replacement. It is, however, important to appreciate that both theoretical predictions and clinical observations indicate that at least 1.5 blood volumes (i.e. 7–8 litres for adults) must be transfused before problems are likely. This will not, however, be true if disseminated intravascular coagulation occurs (see *Coagulation factor depletion* below) or if the patient has pre-existing thrombocytopenia for other reasons.

Platelet counts should be maintained above 50×10^9/l, the minimum level required to achieve effective haemostasis when platelet function is normal. During cardiac bypass surgery, in particular, apparent thrombocytopenic bleeding may occur at counts higher than this, probably because of an acquired functional defect.

Coagulation factor depletion

Despite common assumptions, this is not a frequent occurrence. Stored whole blood contains adequate amounts of all coagulation factors, except for factors V and VIII which decay during storage. Deficiencies even of these factors are less of a problem than supposed. Concentrations of factors V and VIII greater than 20% have, for example, been reported in 21-day stored ACD blood. The synthesis and release of factor VIII also appear to be stimulated by the stress of trauma and surgery. Clearly then, for purely dilutional reasons only mild reductions in total coagulation performance are to be expected following extensive blood loss and stored blood replacement. Disordered haemostasis is more likely to be due to disseminated intravascular coagulation (DIC). This may be revealed by the presence of significantly abnormal laboratory results (for example thrombocytopenia [$< 50 \times 10^9$/l], prolonged prothrombin time and partial thromboplastin time [$> 1.5 \times$ control], hypofibrinogenaemia [< 0.8 g/l] and elevated fibrinogen degradation products) and, in more severe cases, by widespread microvascular bleeding from all cut and injured surfaces. DIC is a likely consequence of delayed or inadequate resuscitation and is probably the explanation for platelet counts and clotting test results that are worse than expected for the volume of transfusion given.

Oxygen affinity changes

Massive rapid transfusion of high oxygen affinity aged stored blood would, on theoretical grounds, be expected to prejudice tissue oxygenation. This, together with the resulting increase in cardiopulmonary workload, could be dangerous in critically ill patients. Although a theoretically convincing case for use of fresh blood can therefore be advanced, objective proof in this clinical setting is hard to come by. While this evidence is awaited it seems reasonable to attempt to use fairly fresh red cell units (e.g. < 1 week old) particularly, for example, where arteriosclerotic vascular disease, or poorly vascularized tissue anastomoses are problems. Absolutely fresh blood (e.g. < 24 hours old) is certainly *not* indicated for this reason alone. It should also be remembered that 2.3 DPG regeneration is a rapid process and recovery of normal oxygen affinity is largely complete within a few hours following transfusion.

Hypocalcaemia

The citrate in anticoagulant fluids binds ionized calcium and potentially lowers plasma calcium levels. This is much less of a problem than might be expected because the healthy adult liver metabolizes citrate at rates equal to 1 unit of blood transfused every 5 minutes. This capacity cannot, however, always be assumed and neonates and hypothermic patients are especially vulnerable to citrate toxicity. Hypocalcaemia does not have a clinically evident effect on blood coagulation; very rarely patients may show a transient tetany. The major consequences of lowered calcium levels are due to its synergism with high potassium levels in disturbing cardiac function (see below). Where clinical and electrocardiographic evidence suggest hypocalcaemia, 5 ml of 10% calcium gluconate (proportionately less for children and neonates) should be given at 5-minute intervals intravenously until the ECG is normal. The advice given formerly that calcium should be administered after transfusion of predetermined amounts of blood is unsafe and unnecessary.

Hyperkalaemia

The plasma potassium content of blood increases during storage and supernatant concentrations may reach over 30 mmol/l. High $K+$ and low $Ca+$ (together with hypothermia and acidosis) combine to impair myocardial performance and could eventually cause cardiac arrest. Hyperkalaemia is in practice not a common problem during transfusion of adults unless large amounts of blood are being given very quickly (hypokalaemia is actually the more frequent finding). Avoidance of hypothermia (see below) is probably the best measure for prevention of effects due to hyperkalaemia and hypocalcaemia.

Acid base disturbances

Lactic acid, the end product of red cell glycolysis in the blood pack, could theoretically contribute to the overall acidosis of hypoxic shocked patients. In practice, however, transfusion usually alleviates acidosis as a result of improved tissue perfusion and relief from hypoxia. The arterial pH should, however, be monitored during massive transfusion. If this cannot be maintained within normal limits by control of pulmonary ventilation and improved perfusion, sodium bicarbonate should be added to intravenous fluids when pH levels fall below 7.2.

Citrate metabolism generates bicarbonate and metabolic alkalosis is the usual consequence of large transfusions.

Hypothermia

Unwanted cooling of the body may result from rapid infusion of blood and other fluids. Blood warmers should be used for rates of infusion exceeding 1 unit per 10 minute in adults and proportionately less for children. Hypothermia slows citrate metabolism, potentiates the harmful cardiac effects of hyperkalaemia and low calcium, and reduces oxygen release from haemoglobin.

Adult respiratory distress syndrome (ARDS)

The aetiology of this condition is not well understood and the importance of various proposed preventive measures remains highly controversial. Certain of the recognized predisposing factors have been mentioned earlier. Under- or over-transfusion should, if possible, be avoided. The plasma oncotic pressure should, if possible, not fall below 20 mmHg (normally associated with serum albumin concentrations below 30 g/l). Hypoproteinaemia will not occur as a result of transfusion unless excessive amounts of crystalloids have been given. If bleeding is continuous, transfusion of whole blood or red cells and plasma is required to prevent development of hypoproteinaemia. Microaggregate filters should be used during massive transfusion except when fresh blood or platelets are administered. The management of established ARDS is beyond the scope of the present chapter.

A management strategy for massive transfusion

Sequence of components

Treat profound hypotension speedily. Prompt administration of any infusion fluid is preferable to delay. In preference order give crystalloids and synthetic colloids (up to 40% blood volume) followed by 4.5% albumin. Initial red cell replacement can take the form of red cell concentrates but, if bleeding continues, it may be more sensible to supply whole blood.

Laboratory samples

At the start blood samples should be collected for blood grouping and cross-matching, coagulation tests and biochemistry profile analysis. These must be properly identified as described in Chapter 12. A fail-safe system must exist for the accurate identification of transfusion samples from emergency admissions.

Blood bank arrangements

The degree of urgency for transfusion should be accurately conveyed to the blood bank.

1 Routine procedures for blood grouping, antibody screening and compatibility testing should be followed as far as practicable unless it is obvious that massive transfusion is likely.

2 If more urgent provision of blood is required this should be clearly indicated by the written request.

3 For extreme emergencies group O blood should be supplied first followed, as soon as possible, by ABO Rh D group specific blood. At the start Rh D negative blood should be used for all women of childbearing age unless this is in such short supply that delays would endanger life. The switch from group O to ABO group specific blood should be made in order to minimize the volume of group O plasma administered. ABO and Rh D matched units can be issued following completion of emergency grouping and an immediate spin saline cross-match against the recipient's serum. It is reasonable to continue transfusing blood on this basis, and later, when time permits, to use the patient's pretransfusion serum to perform an antibody screen. If the antibody screen is negative and more than one blood volume has been exchanged there is no point in attempting compatibility tests apart from performing an immediate spin test to exclude ABO mismatches.

Haematological monitoring

Whenever possible, the investigations shown in Table 17.1 should be performed during massive transfusions. Both the absolute values and the direction of change of results must be considered as a guide to replacement therapy.

Excessive bleeding that does not appear to be due to surgery or trauma should be investigated for evidence of disseminated intravascular coagulation.

Table 17.1 Investigations to be performed during massive transfusions

Investigation	Target value
Haemoglobin; haematocrit	10 g/dl; 0.32
Platelet count	$>50 \times 10^9$/l
Prothrombin time	$<1.5 \times$ control
Partial thromboplastin time	$<1.5 \times$ control
Fibrinogen	>0.8 g/l

Choice of transfusion materials

CRYSTALLOIDS AND COLLOIDS

These are particularly valuable for the initial stage of resuscitation before blood components can be obtained. Isotonic saline and Ringer lactate (compound sodium lactate BP), synthetic colloids (e.g. gelatin, hydroxyethyl starch) and human albumin (4.5%) solution are the principal alternatives; despite extensive studies there is little clinical evidence to support the preferential use of any of these materials. Human albumin should only be used when:

1 two to three litres of crystalloids have already been given, in order to avoid undue reduction of colloid osmotic pressure;

2 patients are known to be hypoproteinaemic with oedema. Human albumin concentrate (20%) must be used where there is a need to increase plasma albumin and colloid osmotic pressures. Target values of 30 g/l and 20 mmHg are usually considered necessary. (One bottle (20 g albumin per 100 ml) should raise plasma albumin by 5–10 g/l in an adult.) Treatment with 4.5% albumin can be recommended for hypotensive episodes not clearly due to recurrent haemorrhage and when the haemoglobin concentration is adequate.

PLATELET CONCENTRATES

Platelet concentrates (1 pack/10 kg) are indicated for continuous (non-surgical) bleeding when platelet counts are below 50×10^9/l or are falling towards that value. There is evidence that platelet functional abnormalities occur in traumatized or massively transfused surgical patients; this phenomenon is certainly well established for cardiac bypass patients. Therapy may, therefore, be justified even at counts between 50 and 100×10^9/l but it is best that supportive evidence in the form of an abnormal standardized template bleeding time be obtained. Each platelet concentrate will also provide around 50 ml fresh plasma!

FRESH FROZEN PLASMA (FFP) OR FRESH FROZEN CRYOSUPERNATANT PLASMA

Frozen plasma (12 ml/kg stat dose or given as 25% of the plasma volume replaced) provides broad spectrum replacement for correction of coagulation abnormalities. Abnormal prothrombin and partial thromboplastin times (e.g. $>1.5\times$ normal or deteriorating) should in theory provide the indications for treatment but in practice these tests correlate poorly with bleeding manifestations. It must also be accepted that although the use of FFP is widely advocated in this context there is still a paucity of objective clinical evidence that it is of any benefit. Continued bleeding together with severely disturbed coagulation tests or laboratory evidence of disseminated intravascular coagulation necessitate more energetic therapy. Platelet concentrates, FFP or, particularly where there is evidence of DIC, cryoprecipitate (1–1.5 packs 10/kg) should be given. Cryoprecipitate will replace fibrinogen and factor VIII in addition to providing von Willebrand factor.

RED CELLS (CONCENTRATES AND OPTIMAL ADDITIVE SUSPENSIONS)

These will be adequate during the initial resuscitation phase but once the need for massive replacement is recognized it is more economical to provide whole blood. Massive transfusion constitutes the only indication for use of this material and in view of the multitude of potential problems faced by the massively haemorrhaging patient (O_2 affinity, plasma K^+, microaggregates) it seems best to ensure that this is not more than 7 days old.

FRESH WHOLE BLOOD

The place of fresh whole blood (e.g. blood donated up to 24 hours previously but still fully tested) in modern transfusion practice is still vigorously contested. Proponents of selective component therapy deny it has any role whilst at the other end of the spectrum there are those (particularly those close to the operating table) who firmly believe that the fresher (and warmer!) the blood is the better.

There is no particular advantage to be gained by transfusing fresh whole blood in these circumstances unless the appropriate components are not readily available.

When to give components

1 For massive uncontrolled traumatic haemorrhage, maintenance of full haemostatic competence by means of component therapy may be unrealistic. In this situation the priority is for major vessel bleeding to be stemmed surgically. Combinations of stored whole blood, red cell concentrates, colloids and crystalloids should be used to maintain blood volume or pressure and haemoglobin or haematocrit values at >7.0 g/dl or 0.25 respectively. It is preferable to conserve use of limited supplies of fresh blood, plasma or platelets until the haemorrhage shows signs of control.

2 When the rate of blood loss is substantially lessened (e.g. 0.5 litres/hour) and after major vessel bleeding is under control, it becomes worthwhile attempting to correct haemostatic abnormalities.

3 Component therapy is particularly indicated where (a) bleeding is presumed to be due to deficient haemostasis rather than from major vessel injuries; this conclusion should be supported by both clinical and laboratory results; and (b) a specific need for components, for example platelets or cryoprecipitate, is disclosed by laboratory results but red cell replacement is not required.

Acknowledgements

During the preparation of this chapter advice was sought from a number of haematologists and specialists in trauma and intensive care, including Professor A.L. Bloom, Dr R.D. Hutton, Dr P. Kernoff, Mr J.S. Spencer, Dr C. Wise, Dr Anne Sutcliffe and Dr C. Thomas. Comments were also sought from the BCSH Haemostasis and Thrombosis Task Force.

Further reading

Bove J.R. (1985) Fresh frozen plasma: too few indications — too much use. *Anesthesia and Analgesia* **64**, 849–850.

Ciavarella D., Reed R.L., Counts R.B., Baron L., Pavlin E., Heimbach D.M. & Carrico J. (1987) Clotting factor levels and the risk of diffuse microvascular bleeding in the massively transfused patient *British Journal of Haematology* **67**, 365–368.

Collins J.A., Murawski K. & Shafer W.A. (eds) (1982) *Massive Transfusion in Surgery and Trauma* Alan R. Liss, New York.

Consensus Conference (1985) Fresh frozen plasma: indications and risks *Journal of the American Medical Association* **253**, 551–553.

Counts R.B., Haisch C., Simon N.G., Maxwell D.M. & Heimbach C.J. (1979) Haemostasis in massively transfused trauma patients. *Annals of Surgery* **190**, 91–99.

International Forum (1976) Fresh blood—a myth or a real need *Vox Sanguinis* **31**, 368–385.

Mannucci P.M., Federici A.B. & Sirchia G. (1982) Hemostasis testing during massive blood replacement. A study of 172 cases *Vox Sanguinis* **42**, 113–123.

Symposium (1984) Management of acute haemorrhage. *Anaesthesia and Intensive Care* **12**, 212–261.

18 Autologous Transfusion

Prepared by the
Blood Transfusion Task Force

General considerations

Autologous transfusion can provide an alternative to using blood from volunteer donors for some patients for elective surgical procedures, avoiding the possibilities of isoimmunization and of acquiring those infections which may be transmitted by a blood transfusion. The guidelines in this chapter relate to blood collected up to 35 days before an elective procedure and stored at 4°C. Pre-deposit of blood to be stored frozen for longer periods is not considered. Directed blood donation, that is donation from relatives or motivated friends of the patient, is not considered and should be actively discouraged since there is no evidence that directed donations are safer than blood provided by the Transfusion Services. Indeed one has to consider that a relative who is in a risk group and under pressure to donate may find it difficult or impossible to avoid doing so.

Autologous transfusion will only be appropriate for a minority of patients; estimates vary depending on several factors of which the more important are the type of patient and surgical procedure studied and the enthusiasm for autologous transfusion of the author of the particular publication. Clearly, the general fitness of the patient to allow several donations to be taken over a short period is of primary importance but other factors such as age, venous access and reliable dates for elective surgery will also be important. Another significant consideration will be the distance from the patient's home to the hospital.

The cost of autologous transfusion in the UK can only be estimated at present and is uncertain.

It has been stated by some advocates of autologous transfusion that it is cheaper than using homologous blood from the Transfusion Services, but this is not immediately obvious as costings need to take account of blood which is collected and not transfused as well as of blood which is used. Costings will also depend on the number and nature of tests performed.

It is recommended that those considering plans to offer autologous transfusion to patients should only do so when appropriate funding has been earmarked and given a priority in their local revenue development programme. Apart from rare medical indications for autologous transfusion (for example, multiple isoantibodies making all donors incompatible) patients having autologous transfusion will do so from preference. In the light of present financial restrictions in the National Health Service, development of autologous transfusion programmes for these patients will almost inevitably be at the expense of some other part of the service.

The advocates of autologous transfusion are concerned to avoid transfusion of homologous blood and it is appropriate to draw attention to other factors which assist in achieving this aim, particularly to the use of haematinics rather than transfusion to raise the haemoglobin where appropriate and to the avoidance of 'one unit' transfusions other than in exceptional circumstances. Equipment designed to salvage shed blood for retransfusion ('cell savers') can also contribute to reducing transfusion requirements. Intraoperative haemodilution may also have a role.

Because autologous transfusion avoids the possibility of isoimmunization or acquisition of disease transmissible by blood transfusion and is therefore regarded as safer in these respects than homologous transfusion, patients being considered for autologous transfusion need to be aware that the procedure has its own inherent risks, particularly those associated with labelling and documentation, and that transposition and transfusion of the wrong blood is a remote but real possibility. A decision to opt for autologous transfusion rather than homologous transfusion is a matter of assessing and balancing the relative risks of the procedures. Patients should be given a realistic picture of the risks which they are seeking to avoid by having autologous transfusion and of the record of very safe transfusion practice based on voluntary donations in the UK.

Selection of patients

Autologous transfusion should only be offered to those patients who would normally be cross-matched for the procedure to be undertaken. Patients who would usually have a 'group and save' should not be considered.

An active bacterial infection is a contraindication to collecting blood for autologous transfusion because of the possibility of bacteraemia which might lead to proliferation of bacteria in stored blood.

Patients suitable for elective surgical procedures who are between the ages of 16 and 65 can be considered, provided that they are free from cardiovascular, cerebrovascular and respiratory disease. Patients over the age of 65 should be considered in the context of their general health since cardiovascular problems increase with age. In young patients, the undesirable effects of several venepunctures on some children need to be considered as the anxiety generated may complicate the induction of anaesthesia for the surgical procedure.

Patients under 7.5 stone (45 kg) need special consideration and it may be appropriate to withdraw smaller volumes than those quoted in Appendix 4.

Patients with a history of fits should not be considered as withdrawal of blood may precipitate an attack.

Patients who have been blood donors and have sustained a delayed faint, i.e. weakness or loss of consciousness several hours after donation, should not be considered.

The patient's haemoglobin should be greater than 12 g/dl in men and 11 g/dl in women. In pregnancy, the haemoglobin should exceed 10 g/dl.

Autologous transfusion can be considered in pregnancy if the patient is fit in other respects and is not suffering from a complication, for example intrauterine growth retardation or pre-eclampsia, which may already have reduced the patient's blood volume (see also Appendix 4).

Selection of patients and consideration of their fitness for the procedure and of the other criteria in this section should be undertaken by the clinician with clinical responsibility for the patient and he/she should also discuss with the patient the relative merits of autologous and homologous transfusion and the possibility that even if autologous transfusion is prepared, it may be necessary to transfuse homologous blood. Nevertheless, the responsibility for ensuring that the patient is in satisfactory health to donate the required number of units rests with the haematologist who agrees to the autologous donations. Referral of suitable patients who wish to have autologous transfusion to the haematologist should be in a standard format signed by the consultant who has discussed autologous transfusion with the patient (Appendix 1).

Practical aspects of collection, storage and transfusion

Collection

Collection and storage of blood for autologous transfusion should be directly supervised by a consultant haematologist. Assuming that the patient has suitable veins and is willing to attend on several occasions, the haematologist should seek the patient's written informed consent to the procedure (Appendix 2) advising the patient about possible complications, particularly the possibility of needing homologous transfusion in addition to any blood prepared for autologous transfusion. The haematologist or a deputed medical officer should be immediately available during blood donation.

Blood collection procedures differ in detail between regions and between regional transfusion centres and hospitals. Important points of procedure can be found in Appendix 4. Consultation with the regional transfusion centre may also be appropriate.

Blood should not be drawn more often than once a week with the last donation a minimum of 4 days (preferably a week) before surgery; this will normally allow up to four or five units to be collected. Exceptionally, for example where surgery is postponed, it may be possible to use a 'leap-frog' technique, returning the oldest unit(s) to the patient to allow another (others) to be withdrawn.

Estimation of the haemoglobin should be carried out before each donation. The haemoglobin should be greater than 12 g/dl in men and 11 g/dl in women before the first procedure and preferably before subsequent donations. Where the haemoglobin is less than 10 g/dl, blood should not be collected.

All patients for autologous transfusion should have a prescription for oral iron.

The label for the blood pack should include the information listed in Appendix 3. The patient should sign the label and should do so immediately before donation, i.e. when the patient is on the couch and after the label has been completed and stuck on the pack. The label should have a suitable adhesive for refrigerated storage.

The following tests should be carried out on the patient.

1 ABO and Rh D—results to be entered on the pack label;

2 Serological screening for atypical antibodies—in case additional homologous blood is required;

3 Tests for HBsAg, anti-HIV and syphilis. These are essential both to establish the patient's status for these markers and because current practices are such that donations which are positive for any of these tests would not be issued for use and the same criteria should apply for autologous transfusion. Advice for the patient about the significance of a positive result in any of these tests should be available.

Storage

Blood for autologous transfusion should be stored in a refrigerator, which is not used for normal blood stocks and cross-matched blood, at a controlled temperature between 4°C and 6°C.

This refrigerator should be equipped with a recorder and an alarm similar to those on other fridges used for blood storage.

Tests pretransfusion

A fresh sample should be obtained from the patient for matching purposes when he/she is admitted for surgery.

The minimum compatibility testing procedure should include ABO and Rh D checks on the patient and on the donations as well as a room temperature 2–5 min spin tube test ('donor' cells × 'patient's' serum), read microscopically.

The standard compatibility testing procedure may integrate better into the routine of most laboratories.

Each donation should carry a compatibility label which is used routinely in the hospital to facilitate checking in theatre and at the bedside. Design of the autologous transfusion label should allow the compatibility label to be overstuck leaving the information about the blood group and expiry date readily visible.

Disposal of unused blood

Blood collected for autologous transfusion which is not required for the donating patient must not be transfused to another patient. Blood for autologous transfusion which is not transfused may be used for laboratory purposes, provided that HBsAg and anti-HIV tests have been carried out. Otherwise unused blood must be discarded. Plasma from unused blood should not be included in pools for fractionation. The fate of autologous blood should be fully documented to ensure that each unit can be accounted for (circular C/84(7)).

Quality control

A proportion of donations collected for autologous transfusion should be cultured for possible contaminating micro-organisms. This can be most easily achieved by culturing some or all, depending on numbers, of the unused donations. At least 1% of blood collected should be cultured by both aerobic and anaerobic techniques.

Appendix 1: Referral letter to consultant haematologist

Dear

This patient has requested autologous transfusion for his/her operation. I have discussed this with the patient, with appropriate reference to *Guidelines for autologous transfusion* and am of the opinion that he/she is medically suitable for the procedure.

I would be grateful if you would see him/her with a view to making the necessary arrangements.

Patient's name (Mr/Mrs/Ms): ....

Patient's address: ....

....

Patient's date of birth: ....

Ward: ....

Hospital: ....

Hospital number: ....

Date of admission: ....

Date of operation: ....

Planned procedure: ....

Underlying pathology: ....

Requested number of donations (maximum is 5): ....

Haemoglobin (g/dl): ....

Signature of referring consultant clinician: ....

Name of referring consultant clinician (BLOCK LETTERS): ....

Date: ....

Appendix 2: Consent to autologous transfusion

The purpose of autologus transfusion has been explained to me by Dr ....
who has also explained its possible complications and hazards.

I agree to my blood being withdrawn and stored for autologous transfusion.

I understand that it may not be possible for technical reasons to return to me all or any of the units which I donate.

I understand that it may be necessary to supplement my autologous transfusion with blood from volunteer donors from the Transfusion Services.

I agree to my blood being tested for HBsAg (one of the viruses causing hepatitis) and for anti-HIV (the virus associated with AIDS) and syphilis.

Signed ....

Dated ....

Witnessed ....

Appendix 3: Blood pack label

Blood for autologous transfusion should be identified with an overstick label* which includes the following information:

BLOOD FOR AUTOLOGOUS TRANSFUSION ONLY

Surname
First names
Date of birth
Hospital number
Date of collection
Date of expiry
ABO and Rh (D) types
Lab. ref. number
Patient's signature

The patient signs the pack to confirm that the details on the label (apart from the ABO and (D) type which may not be entered when the first unit is drawn) are correct. The signature can also be compared as part of a pretransfusion checking procedure with the signature on the consent form which by then will be in the patient's notes.

Appendix 4: Blood collection

The following points are of importance in collecting a blood donation.

*This label should not occlude the information given on the manufacturer's standard pack label.

1 Check the patient's blood pressure.

2 Collect blood into a single pack with CPD-A1 anticoagulant to give a shelf-life of 35 days.

3 Use a balance to measure the volume of blood drawn.

4 The skin should be cleaned thoroughly using chlorhexidine (in alcohol) or equivalent.

5 The use of local anaesthetic is recommended.

6 The donor tubing should be clamped, for example with 'non-toothed' Spencer Wells forceps, before the guard is removed from the needle. This will prevent air entering the bag and possibly contaminating the donation. The clamp should remain in place until after the venepuncture.

7 A normal donation should be approximately 450 ml, but a smaller volume may be appropriate. Packs for the collection of 250 ml are available.

8 The pack should be agitated gently throughout collection to mix the blood with the anticoagulant.

9 Samples for laboratory tests can be taken at the end of the donation before the needle is withdrawn by clamping the donor tube in two places and cutting the tube between the clamps.

10 Attention to haemostasis after withdrawal of the needle will be particularly important if several donations need to be collected from the vein.

11 It is important to use a roller stripper to evacuate the blood from the donor tube into the pack and allow it to be replaced with anticoagulated blood.

12 The donor tube should be sealed, both at its cut end and close to the pack.

Note: pregnant patients

In the latter part of pregnancy, the weight of the uterus in the dorsal position impedes venous return. Because of this, these patients are more likely to react adversely to venesection and donations should therefore be collected with the patient lying in the lateral position.

Appendix 5: Fact sheet

This fact sheet provides information for patients. Additions or amendments, taking account of local practices, may be needed.

FACTS ABOUT AUTOLOGOUS BLOOD TRANSFUSION

What is autologous blood?

Autologous blood is blood from an individual to be given back to that individual should the need for transfusion arise. Blood can be stored for up to 35 days between collection and use.

What are the advantages of autologous blood?

Autologous blood has the advantage over blood from other individuals in that it is incapable of stimulating antibodies to red cells, white cells, platelets and plasma proteins.

It also carries no risk of transmitting infections such as hepatitis or AIDS. However, the very small risk of bacterial contamination at the time of collection is the same as for any blood donation.

What are the disadvantages of autologous blood?

In general, donation for autologous transfusion has the same minimal risk as any blood donation. Because of the need to collect several units of blood within a period of a few weeks, it will be necessary for the patient to take an iron supplement. There is also a minimal risk that blood other than one's own may be transfused accidentally.

Who may donate for autologous transfusion?

Patients between the ages of 16 and 65, and some older patients whose general health is good, can be considered for autologous transfusion for some planned surgical and obstetric procedures. The consultant in charge of your case will decide if you are suitable for autologous transfusion.

How many units of autologous blood may be donated?

The exact number would be determined by your consultant. As many as four or five units may be taken at approximately weekly intervals before the planned date for surgery.

Where is blood donated?

The donations will be taken at your local hospital or regional transfusion centre. The request is made by your consultant to the haematologist who will arrange to collect and store your donations.

How long does the procedure take?

Collecting a donation takes about 30 minutes each time, after which you will be asked to rest for 15 minutes before leaving. You can drive a car afterwards if you feel perfectly well, but it may be advisable to have a friend who is willing to drive on the first visit. If you feel unwell or if you are in any doubt, you should inform the haematologist. Some occupations involve some personal risks or include responsibility for the safety of others. If such hazards are a normal part of your work, ask the haematologist how long you should wait before resuming your activities.

POINTS TO NOTE AFTER THE DONATION

1 Most people feel fine after donating; however, if you do feel light-headed it may mean that your system has not had enough time to adjust. You should restrict your activities and, if necessary, lie down and rest until you feel better.

2 Drinking extra fluid helps to replace some of the liquid portion of the blood you have donated. You will normally be offered a drink following donation.

3 If your arm starts to bleed, do not be alarmed. Simply raise the arm above your head and apply gentle continuous pressure immediately to the venepuncture for 10 or 15 minutes until bleeding stops.

4 Occasionally the area may appear bruised. This discoloration will disappear within a few days and should cause you no concern.

5 Usually the venepuncture heals without difficulty. However, if the site should become reddened and painful, you should contact the haematologist or your general practitioner.

19 Product Liability for the Hospital Blood Bank

Prepared by the Blood Transfusion Task Force

Introduction

In 1985 a European Community Directive was produced to the effect that all Member States must have strict civil liability laws to cover damage caused by defective products. In the UK this led to the Consumer Protection Act of 1987 and in particular to Part 1 of the Act which covers product liability and came into force on 1 March 1988. Prior to this legislation if a consumer came to harm as a result of a defective product it was necessary to prove negligence on the part of the producer in order to win a case for damages. The new legislation removes the need to prove negligence—it is sufficient to prove that the product was defective and resulted in damage to the consumer. Compensation can be sought for death, personal injury or damage to private property.

In addition to manufactured substances, those which have been 'won' or 'abstracted' are included in the definition of a 'product'. It has been determined that blood is such a product. The regional centres of the Transfusion Service and the Plasma Fractionators are readily identified as the main 'producers' of blood and blood products, although other participants in the chain of supply between the producer and the consumer have been identified with liabilities and responsibilities of their own. Hospital blood banks readily fit this role of intermediary and can even, in certain circumstances, be considered the 'producer' of the product. It is more likely, however, that the hospital blood bank will be seen as the *supplier* of a product to the patient or the *keeper* of equipment.

Chain of product supply

In order to bring an action against a producer the consumer will obviously approach the supplier to trace/identify the producer. If the supplier cannot identify the producer then liability rests with the supplier, i.e. 'the buck stops'. The threat of such a penalty demands the keeping of accurate records, to be immediately available on request.

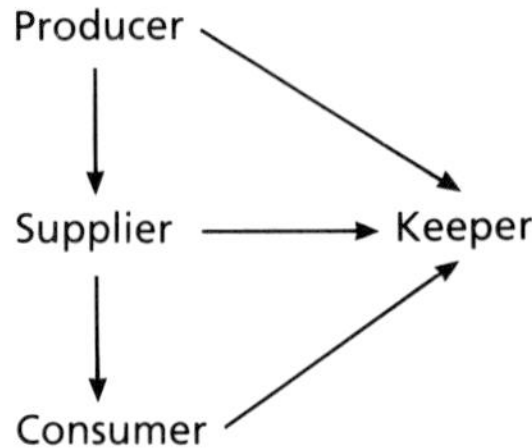

There are defences open to the producer under the Act. The most controversial is the 'Development Risks' or 'State of the Art' defence which is allowed under UK legislation, but excluded in the legislation taken by several other EC members. This defence is however not likely to impinge on hospital blood banks. Likely to be of much more significance is the defence that the defect was not in the product at the time of supply, i.e. it arose in the hands of the supplier.

The requirement for the supplier to identify the producer and to ensure that defects do not originate whilst products are in the hands of the supplier illustrates the need for hospital blood banks to grasp the nettle of Product Liability Legislation and the resulting implications for routine working practices.

The hospital blood bank

General

The aim of those involved in transfusion medicine/science is to provide the patient with an effective product, which achieves maximum therapeutic effect with minimum risk. It is unlikely that such a biological source material as blood will ever allow the production of entirely risk-free and defect-free products. Our energies are rather directed towards reducing the risk to a minimum. One current approach within the Transfusion Service is via the implementation of Quality Assurance systems to cover and improve all the steps involved in the production of its products, from donor to patient. In addition to the quality of the raw materials such systems encompass the quality of premises, storage, equipment, reagents, staff selection, training and continuing education. For such systems to be successful they cannot grind to a halt at the blood bank door—they must be continued through to the bedside and involve the Hospital Transfusion Committee. Recommended standards for blood bank procedures exist on many levels from international (World Health Organization, Council of Europe), through national (American Association of Blood Banks, joint British Blood Transfusion Society/British Society for Haematology, Joint NBTS/NIBSC), to local in-house standards. Such standards tend to become more demanding as their intended sphere of influence contracts. In devising targets however it is essential that they remain realistic and achievable otherwise the result will be demoralized staff rather than increased quality of working practice. Participation in external quality control systems is essential.

The fact that procedures and products can be shown to comply with recognized standards is not an absolute defence; however, it is likely that such compliance would be looked on favourably and might limit the damages awarded. Lack of compliance with existing recognized standards could only worsen the situation.

Standard operating procedures (See Appendices)

It is essential that every activity, whether routine or rare, carried out within the blood bank should have a documented, defined standard operating procedure (SOP). *An SOP for a given procedure should enable any competent worker to follow the procedure.* It should define the materials and equipment required and point out any hazards or pitfalls of the procedure. This should then be followed by a clear, albeit apparently pedantic, step-by-step, description of the procedure. Reference to related SOPs should be made.

Such SOPs should be regularly reviewed and updated as details change. It should be a 'live' document referred to regularly and be reflected in the working practices of the laboratory. It should not be regarded as an unrealistic statement of the ideal and gather dust in a cupboard.

All members of staff working within the blood bank, especially those performing only on-call duties, should be familiar with the contents of the department SOPs. They are important in the induction and training of new members of staff who, with other staff, should not only read the SOPs, but sign to that effect after they have been trained in the practice described by the SOP.

The compilation of SOPs may be laborious and time consuming, but once generated they provide clarity, definition and consistency to a given process.

The place of the blood bank in the supply chain

Blood and its products are easily identified as 'products' covered by the Act when received by the hospital blood bank. There is little doubt that the blood bank then fulfils the role of *supplier.*

Blood banks use equipment such as refrigerators, freezers, water-baths, centrifuges and automated cell washing centrifuges for antiglobulin tests (IAT) in the provision of their services to the patient. They are the *keeper* of such equipment. They also use external manufacturers' reagents and tests kits.

In certain circumstances the blood bank could be considered the *producer.*

The blood bank as *supplier*

The blood bank assumes the role of supplier of blood products on receipt of products from the transfusion service. Without exception this will be accompanied by documentation, the accuracy of which must be checked and the information stored.

It is the responsibility of the producer to provide recommendations with respect to maintenance, expiry dates and conditions of storage of their products. It is the responsibility of the supplier to adhere to these recommendations and to provide recorded evidence that these conditions have been met. Such recommendations should be passed to the user at time of onward supply.

Rigid adherence to manufacturers' or producers' instructions is vital. If instructions have not been followed then this may at best be considered contributory negligence and the liability be shared with the producer. At worst such deviation from instructions may be considered sufficient to break the chain of responsibility, releasing the producer and leaving the laboratory to bear full liability.

It appears inevitable that the principle role of the supplier will be in record keeping. In the event of a patient suffering as a result of a blood product shown to have been defective the blood bank must be able to provide evidence identifying the producer. It is insufficient to say that 'we always get all our blood from Centre X' or 'all our albumin comes from Company Y'. Records must be kept for all products to show clearly from whom and when a product was obtained and to whom and when it was supplied. Product batch numbers must be recorded. It must be possible to trace *all* blood products transfused to an individual patient.

A court action under the Act must begin within 3 years of awareness of injury and within 10 years of the date of supply by the producer. Thus hospital blood banks are advised to keep records for at least 11 years (15 years at transfusion centres). This has significant implications in terms of staff time and data storage. Many are taking advantage of new technology data handling and storage systems. It should be remembered that such systems may have significant cost implications.

The blood bank is responsible for ensuring and providing evidence of the correct conditions of storage for blood and products. Standards exist for blood bank blood refrigerators (BS 4376) and it is recommended that the temperature be controlled at $4°C \pm 2°C$. Such dedicated refrigerators should have a graphic temperature recorder and an audible alarm with a back-up battery power supply. A remote alarm should register at a central area such as the hospital switchboard when the department is not staffed. Freezers should also have graphic temperature recorders and audible alarms.

It is recommended that blood banks retain responsibility for satellite blood storage refrigerators, for example within theatre suites. Such refrigerators should comply with blood bank refrigerator standards and their use covered by an SOP.

When blood is transferred between hospitals it is in the interests of the receiving hospital to ensure that it has been stored under correct conditions in the supplying hospital. It would be prudent and not unreasonable to request written confirmation of satisfactory prior storage conditions.

The blood bank as *keeper*

If a patient suffers as a result of faulty 'equipment', for example a defective Coombs washer or faulty reagent purchased by the blood bank, then the liability rests with the producer or supplier of the equipment. However, this may pass to the blood bank, the keeper of the equipment, if it can be shown that the equipment has not been maintained, calibrated or used in accordance with instructions.

A system of planned preventative maintenance should be introduced and regular calibration or performance checks should be undertaken. Again records of maintenance and calibration should be kept. It is obvious that equipment should be kept clean, both for the health and safety of the staff and to avoid contamination of blood products. Particular attention should, for example, be paid to water-baths used for thawing fresh frozen plasma and cryoprecipitate. The liability for a unit of FFP contaminated with a pseudomonad from a water-bath will rest neither with the 'producer'—the defect did not exist at the time of supply—nor with the manufacturer of the water-bath.

It is not unusual for laboratories to have equipment on trial. The position of such 'loan' equipment is unclear, but it has been suggested that as no formal purchase has been made the equipment might be considered at law to be covered by the rules of charity and the manufacturer/lender could not be held liable for the consequences of any defect. It would be wise to consider this before accepting equipment on trial and to seek a written agreement from the lender accepting liability for defects.

Blood banks buy significant amounts of reagents, panels and test kits. All include detailed package inserts with instructions for use. If, in the event of damage it can be shown that the recommended instructions were not followed then the manufacturer and supplier can escape liability which will then devolve on the laboratory concerned. If any deviation from recommended technique is to be introduced its effect on the results obtained must be fully validated prior to its introduction. The laboratory then assumes responsibility for the procedure, and the documentation of such validation must be available for inspection.

The blood bank as *producer*

The producer (i) manufactures the product; or (ii) wins or abstracts it; or (iii) carries out a process to which essential characteristics of the product are attributable.

If the goods do not originate within the European Community (EC) then liability rests with the original importer of the goods into the Community. Note should be taken of the country of origin of imported equipment. Hospital-based donations of blood and blood components may involve the blood bank as a producer under (i) and (ii). Under (iii) above does the hospital blood bank which uses laboratory-based leucocyte depleting filters to produce leucocyte poor blood for example alter the 'essential' characteristics of the product to the extent that they now bear the mantle of 'producer'? There is no definitive answer as yet—we await the evolution of case law to set precedents. In the meantime any blood bank performing such manipulations on blood or its products should ensure that the efficacy and sterility of their procedure is fully validated and documented.

Liability for defective products can also rest with 'any person, who by putting his name on the product, or using a trade mark or other distinguishing mark in relation to the product, has held himself out to be the producer of the product'. Where does that leave the blood bank cross-matching labels? Current advice is that the label should not obscure the information concerning the origin of the unit of blood or precautions regarding storage and use and that its content be confined to essential factual information. Attention should be paid to the adhesive properties of cross-match labels at 4°C when adhesion should be optimal.

Documentation

Reference should be made to the BCSH 'Guidelines for hospital blood bank documentation and procedure' (see Chapter 12).

It is clear that product liability legislation will lead to an increase in the quantity and quality of documentation surrounding the use of blood and blood products and that there will be significant cost implications.

The 'producers' have to ensure that their package inserts are comprehensive but understandable. The suppliers have to follow the instructions and ensure that they are passed on to the user.

Blood banks must keep full, detailed and meticulous records of product receipt and release and maintenance records to cover equipment.

It is well known that most incompatible transfusions are the result of clerical and not serological error. The hospital blood bank laboratory has always been most insistent on sample labelling, the accompanying forms being complete, and patient identity unambiguous. The current legislation further justifies such an approach and blood banks should continue to explore new developments in patient identification systems in order to increase the security of their documentation.

In future laboratories will have to pay significantly more attention to the wording of supply agreements/contracts for the products they purchase. The small print must be scrutinized and any attempts to transfer liability from manufacturer to user via indemnity clauses resisted. Indemnity clauses may not in any case be valid under this legislation, but it will be simpler not to accept them in the first place than to argue the point at a later date.

The consumer—in this case the patient—cannot waive his/her rights under this legislation. There is no future in forms waiving those rights even though signed by the patients—such forms have no legal standing at all and serve only to worry and deceive the patients.

Conclusion

There are many points on product liability which will only be clarified with the evolution of case law. In the meantime we must do what we can. The ultimate beneficiary of product liability legislation is the consumer. It was not designed to make life more complicated for the laboratory, although the increased documentation and data storage in order to defend an action which may take a decade to arise, if at all, may be cumbersome. The positive side to the legislation will be in forcing blood banks to confront the need for an active Quality Assurance system, the benefits from which will be apparent in the short term. After all we share with the legislators the desire to deliver the safest possible product to the patients.

Appendix 1: Standard operating procedures (SOPs)

Any document published on a local, regional or national basis must, in the light of present trends, have a legal implication if it affects the issue of a result or product to a patient.

The increase in medical litigation demands the production of a manual of information and methodology by every department undertaking work in the field of transfusion science, both as a point of reference and as a safeguard for those staff in the face of possible litigation.

In compiling an SOP, its legal position should be considered as having the same importance as its content.

CONTENT

General information

As many staff only work in the transfusion department during the course of 'on-call' duties, it is essential that general information includes such items as procedures to be followed in the event of a blood bank alarm activation, or, if the department is computerized, the procedure to be followed in the event of a major computer crash. Those procedures that are carried out infrequently must also be listed. It is also advisable to keep any published documents, for example DoH safety booklets, in close proximity to the SOP for immediate referral when required.

SOPs should be written by the most senior staff actually performing the duties or functions. Initial drafts should record faithfully what is actually happening —not what should happen or what looks good on paper. This draft must be corrected, where necessary, to reflect what should be happening, and unacceptable practices changed immediately. The head of the department or supervisor should vet the SOP and prior to final acceptance it should be scrutinized by a small committee, including the person who produced the document, taking into account GMP and health and safety requirements.

Methodology

All methodology in use in a department must be written down in good, well punctuated English, devoid of ambiguities. It is advisable that attention should be given to any published guidelines which document methodologies currently approved. It is essential that the document does not contain misinformation.

Each SOP issued must be accounted for and a careful note taken of persons or departments receiving copies, who must sign for them (Appendix 3). Unauthorized copies are not permitted. Some method should be devised to ensure staff are using the current edition, for example stamping each page with the comment 'OFFICIAL SOP if stamped RED'. It is better to issue extra copies which can be accounted for than have staff photocopy for their personal use.

For ease of maintaining an update facility, it is recommended that the SOP should be kept on a word processor disc. This obviates the necessity for major rewriting for minor alterations in a method.

All official copies of SOPs must be accounted for and destroyed before issue of a new version, but a master copy of all superseded SOPs should be kept for reference purposes by the head of the Quality Assurance Department, or by the overall head of department if no Quality Assurance Department yet exists.

LEGAL IMPLICATIONS OF AN SOP

Implications for the author/compiler

The individual who draws up an SOP clearly should do so in a professional manner, with regard both to all those likely to be affected by it, and to his or her employer.

In practice, where a Health Authority employee may become personally liable for a claim in negligence (for example by a patient) for actions carried out while at work, the Authority provides a complete indemnity. It is extremely rare for individual members of staff to be sued personally.

So far as responsibilities to the employer are concerned, the obligation is similar, and short of deliberate misinformation no problem is likely to arise.

Effect of adopting a standard procedure

The object of having a standard procedure is to eliminate potentially harmful or dangerous alternative methods. Whether or not the Authority would wish to make a failure to comply a disciplinary matter is up to them. In our view a persistent failure should be regarded as serious, but it may be more appropriate for minor isolated breaches to be dealt with informally and followed up with appropriate retraining.

If any breach is to be regarded as a disciplinary matter then this should be made clear to staff; otherwise the position is that the Authority would approach the matter on the basis of a breach of professional standards amounting to misconduct and the SOP would be relevant as evidence of what the professional level of competence should be.

The effect of litigation with third parties

An SOP is of value as evidence when dealing with claims where negligence is alleged in patient care covered by the procedure. If the action criticized by the patient is in accordance with a standard procedure, it is difficult for a judge to find that the action was negligent, and the force of this is greater the wider the procedure is agreed. Conversely a failure to comply with a standard procedure is likely to attract a finding of negligence unless there are compelling reasons for having adopted that course.

These considerations are very much less relevant in the context of product liability under the Consumer Protection Act. Such liability is strict, subject to certain limitation, and if blood supplied to a patient is 'defective' (e.g. infected) then in general it is no defence to say that the SOPs were complied with. However, the procedure may be relevant (although not conclusive) to establish the state of scientific and technical knowledge at the relevant time, if the 'State of the Art' defence is relied upon.

Where in effect there is a national (or European) standard which is adopted and modified for individual hospitals or districts, it is important to keep a record of the reasons for any modification.

A SUMMARY GUIDELINE FOR THE PREPARATION OF AN SOP

An SOP contains an accurate written description of a working procedure and must comply with good manufacturing practice (see p. 226). The preparation of an SOP is the responsibility of the head of the section as it is one of the means of managerial control.

It must include the sections outlined below.

1 A clear, brief title and a unique document identity number.

2 A brief description of the purpose of the procedure.

3 An outline of the principle on which the procedure is based.

4 Specification of

(a) Staff, qualifications, experience and training.

(b) Reagents, equipment and protocols in the order in which they should be used and the location of these items in the laboratory.

5 Health and safety notes must include any specific hazards and their handling procedures. (Brief notes and references to appropriate documents.)

6 The SOP procedure should be given in numbered steps which logically follow the working procedure, and are written in simple, unambiguous language in the imperative (must or shall, not should or may).

Main points to consider in the preparation of an SOP

1 If the procedure is carried out in two or more stages, divide the SOP into separate sections. Provide an index to the sections at the top of the procedure.

2 If *any part* of the procedure uses a commercial kit, then the reader may be directed to the manufacturer's instructions to ensure that the product liability borne by the manufacturer is maintained. The relevant information should be photocopied and attached to the SOP.

3 Copies of forms used in the procedure should be listed with the details of equipment and attached to the SOP.

4 An example form clearly marked EXAMPLE may be attached to the SOP to clarify a procedure.

5 Before approving an SOP, a senior person and one or two routine staff should try out the procedure given by the SOP.

6 It is useful if the SOP can be compiled on a word processor to facilitate simple modifications.

7 The SOP must be approved by an independent senior person, expert in the procedure, if a quality assurance officer is not available. This is essential to ensure that the SOP meets the requirements of the *Guide to Good Manufacturing Practice*, relevant Acts of Parliament and Health and Safety documents.

8 When the SOP is finalized it must be signed by the head of department and the date of approval placed on the top of each page of the document.

9 In addition to the date of approval the top of each page of an SOP must carry the unique identification and page numbers.

10 Record the date of issue of an SOP in an SOP issue file and, when an SOP is updated, withdraw all obsolete copies apart from one reference copy in the SOP file. Record the dates of revision and approval.

11 A copy of the SOP must be readily available in the department where the procedure is carried out.

MAJOR REFERENCES TO BE CONSULTED IN PREPARATION OF SOPS

HMSO Publications

1 *Guide to Good Pharmaceutical Manufacturing Practice*, HMSO 1983 (previous issues of this Guide 1971, 1977 may also prove useful).
2 *Categorization of pathogens according to hazards and categories of containment*, Advisory Committee on Dangerous Pathogens, London HMSO 1984.

British Standards

1 BS 5750 Part II 1987, Quality Systems.
2 BS 4402, 1982, Safety Requirements for Laboratory Centrifuges.

Acts of Parliament

1 Health and Safety at Work Act etc. 1974 Chapter 37.

2 Consumer Protection Act 1987, particularly Part I.
3 Guide to the Consumer Protection Act 1987; Product Liability and Safety Provisions. (Department of Trade and Industry.)
4 Control of Substances Hazardous to Health Regulations 1988.

DoH publications/circulars/notices

1 *HSAC: Safety in Health Service Laboratories: Safe Working and the Prevention of Infection in Clinical Laboratories*, 1990.
2 Health Equipment Information, *Management of Equipment* Number 98, January 1982.
3 DHSS Health Notice, *Product Liability* HN88 (3), March 1988.
4 *Good Laboratory Practice: The United Kingdom Compliance Programme*, 1989.

Other documents

1 Health and Safety Handbook IND (G) 37 (L), *Working with VDUs.*
2 *Guidelines for the Blood Transfusion Services in the United Kingdom* (1989/90).

Appendix 2: Example of a 'policy' SOP

DISCREPANT BLOOD GROUP

Procedures to be followed when a discrepancy is found in the results of blood grouping on samples purported to be from the same patient.

Antenatal and pre-operative samples

The requesting clinician must be informed of the discrepancy and further samples *must* be submitted for testing. Under no circumstances must a report be issued until repeat samples have been tested. The matter must be referred to the consultant haematologist for reporting.

Samples for cross-matching

Non-urgent—the medical officer in charge of the patient must be contacted and further samples requested. If there is any resistance to this request, the consultant haematologist or haematologist 'on-call' must be contacted for advice.

Urgent or life-threatening situations

The medical officer in charge of the patient must be informed of the discrepancy and further samples requested. If there is any resistance to this request, the consultant haematologist must be contacted for advice. If this is not possible, group O Rhesus negative blood must be issued until a further sample is received for confirmation of the patient's group. The medical officer in charge of the patient should be informed of the risks of this course of action.

Appendix 3: Sample method of document control

Glasgow and West of Scotland
Regional Transfusion Centre

Standard operating procedure

No:
Supersedes no:
No. of pages:

1 Title:

2 Area(s) of application:

3 Discussed by SOP Review Committee on:

Accepted for issue: Revision required:

Authorized by: Date:

4 Number of copies issued:

Section	No. of copies	Issued by	Received by	Date

CONFIDENTIAL

Note: The production of unauthorized copies is not permitted

5 Destruction of copies ______________ Recovered and destroyed by ________

on __________________________ Copies missing __________________

Further investigation required/not required

Signed ________________________ Date ________________________

Appendix 4: Example of an 'operative' SOP

Borchester Royal Infirmary Haematology Department
Standard Operating Procedure
Temperature monitoring of blood storage refrigerators

SOP No. 01/01 Blood Bank

Areas of application:
- Blood bank
- Blood bank refrigerators in operating theatre suite and obstetric delivery suite.

This document comprises three pages and is only valid if each page is endorsed with the official SOP stamp in red ink. A member of staff may only perform this task if authorized to do so by the blood bank Chief MLSO.

Prepared by .... Authorized by ....
(*Section Head*) (*Head of Department*)

Date ....

[Page 1 ends here]

Temperature monitoring of blood storage refrigerators

Introduction
Red cell components must at all times be stored refrigerated at 4° ±2°C. Storage temperatures must be monitored continuously and a permanent record produced. An alarm system, giving warning of temperature deviations must provide a signal at a continuously staffed site.

Principle of the procedure
The temperature monitoring system utilizes sensors (a) in air to measure refrigerator air temperature surrounding the blood units and (b) in water to provide an indication of the likely temperature of blood units. This latter sensing element is connected to a recording thermograph giving a continuous paper record.

Audible and visible alarms must warn of air temperature changes beyond the limits of 1.5–8.5°C and power failure. Technical details can be obtained from BS 4376 specification for electrically operated blood storage refrigeration.

Personnel
Staff will carry out refrigeration temperature checks at the direction of the blood bank CMLSO.

Equipment
Installations to be monitored comprise:
1 uncross-matched blood refrigerator (No. 1) located in the blood bank;
2 cross-matched blood refrigerator (No. 2) located in the blood bank;
3 blood storage refrigerator (No. 3) located in the annexe to main theatre suite;
4 blood bank storage refrigerator (No. 4) located in obstetric delivery suite.

Procedure

1 Daily inspections.

(a) Examine thermograph recorder charts to ensure that the temperature has not exceeded the limits 2–6 °C.

[Page 2 ends here]

(b) Confirm that the digital reading of air temperature agrees with the minimax thermometer situated in the main refrigerator compartment.

(c) Sign charts to confirm that the inspection has been carried out and that the temperature has been maintained correctly.

(d) Report any discrepancies between thermometer and thermograph readings or deviations from stated temperature limits immediately to the blood bank CMLSO or deputy.

2 Weekly checks:

(a) These must be carried out each Thursday.

(b) Change the 7 day chart recorder paper and rewind the recorder clock mechanism.

(c) Write the refrigerator number and the day's date on the back of the recorder chart and file it.

(d) Test local and remote alarm systems by moving the recorder pens above and below the preset limits.

(e) Test local and remote alarms for power failure.

(f) Notify the blood bank CMLSO or deputy immediately in the event of malfunction.

3 Instructions for dealing with malfunction of alarms or refrigeration systems are provided in SOP 01/02 (blood bank) and SOP 01/03 (blood bank) respectively.

Health and safety requirements

None applicable to temperature monitoring.

Procedure for dealing with blood spillage is covered by SOP 01/04 (blood bank).

Reference

BS 4376 1982 for blood bank refrigeration (currently undergoing revision).

20 Clinical Use of Blood Cell Separators

Prepared by the
Clinical Haematology Task Force

Introduction

These guidelines replace the DHSS *Code of practice for the clinical use of blood cell separators* (1977) and supplement the *Guidelines for the use of automated machine plasma and platelet apheresis of volunteer donors within the UK blood transfusion service* (1985).

The guidelines apply both to patients and donors. Patient procedures include:

1 plasma exchange with or without absorption columns or secondary membranes; and

2 cytapheresis procedures which remove red cells, white cells or platelets.

Donor procedures include:

1 white cell donation;

2 platelet donation; and

3 plasma donation in excess of 600 ml with plasma substitute replacement.

The potential complications of therapeutic cell separator procedures are set out in Appendix 1.

The clinical criteria that apply are inevitably not the same as those for volunteer donors set out in the document *Guidelines for the use of automated machine plasma and platelet apheresis of volunteer donors within the UK blood transfusion service.*

When considering the siting of a cell separator, it should be remembered that the equipment should be used regularly and frequently (i.e., on average at least twice a week), so that staff can maintain a high standard of proficiency in the operation and care of this equipment.

Clinical management of the cell separator service

A consultant, who will normally be a haematologist, must be in overall charge. The consultant is responsible for advice concerning cell separator procedures and for determining which patients and donors are suitable for these procedures, having regard to safety and to the general condition of the patient or donor. The consultant or his/her deputy is responsible for assessing patients and donors prior to the procedure and it follows that the patient should be referred to the consultant for determining which investigations are to be undertaken. The consultant or a medical deputy appointed by him/her should normally be present at the commencement of a procedure and must remain in the vicinity until the completion of the procedure. Patients and donors should never be left in a room without the attendance of a registered nurse or doctor.

Patients

Informed consent

While it is not necessary to obtain written consent from patients (in normal circumstances the patient's attendance implies consent), it is important to ensure that whenever a patient's condition allows, a full explanation of the procedure is given by a doctor competent in cell separation procedures. In obtaining verbal consent, the doctor must explain the purpose of the separation, describe the procedure and explain the possible risks and discomfort involved. It is imperative that details of this consultation are recorded in the casenotes and signed by the doctor in attendance.

Examination of patients

The doctor in charge of the procedure must ensure that there are no medical contraindications to the performance of the procedure and in particular must see that the patient's pulse, blood pressure and cardiorespiratory status have been recorded in the case notes. Where the patient is not under the continuing care of the doctor using the separator, a record of formal examination is required. If there are plans to use any material obtained from patients, agreement must first be obtained for hepatitis B antigen and HIV screening (see below).

Frequency and volume of apheresis

The consequences of multiple apheresis must be considered whenever recurrent procedures are required. Few medical conditions require more than 5 consecutive days' apheresis and usually fewer procedures are necessary during the first week of treatment. The volume of plasma removed should be related to the patient's estimated plasma volume. Each procedure normally involves a 1–1.5 times plasma volume exchange, which in an adult usually involves a 2–4 litre exchange per procedure. Very occasionally apheresis is needed in children and it is essential that the volume of plasma removed is appropriately reduced to take account of the smaller plasma volume. A worksheet should be kept of the details of each procedure. Special note must be made of any adverse patient reactions.

See Appendix 2 for operational guidelines defining the standards of care required.

Donors

Selection and care of donors

Donors should be accepted according to the advice given in the National Blood Transfusion Service memorandum on the selection, medical examination and care of blood donors (1984) with the exception that the higher age limit should normally be 55 years. First-time donors should not normally be accepted over the age of 50 years or under 50 kg in weight and they should preferably have given two routine blood donations without untoward effects. Occasionally first-time donors may be accepted if they are specifically motivated, for example friend, relative or hospital volunteers, but they must fulfil the remaining criteria. Normally, unrelated donors should be recruited from the National Blood Transfusion Service donor panels and requests for unrelated donors should be made to the regional transfusion director.

For platelet donations, the donor should not have taken any aspirin or other platelet-active drugs for an appropriate period. For aspirin, this is about 7 days, but for other drugs this may be shorter.

Care must be taken to ensure that undue pressure is not put on persons to donate, particularly if they are related to the patient or are an HLA matched donor. Donors must not be placed in a position where it is difficult for them not to continue making further donations although they wish to stop.

Where a patient or a relative is acting as a donor and fails to meet the standard criteria, their donor eligibility must be reviewed by the consultant in charge of the unit.

Before a volunteer is enrolled as a member of a cell separator donor panel, his/her general practitioner should preferably be consulted.

Informed consent

A consent form must be signed by each donor prior to the donation (see Appendix 3) and this must include consent for anti-HIV and HB_sAg screening. Before giving written consent, the volunteer should be fully informed about the procedure he/she will undergo and the risks incurred, by the doctor in charge of the procedure. In obtaining informed consent, the donor should be given the following information.

1 The purpose of the donation.

2 A description of the proposed procedure and the likely duration of the donation.

3 A description of the risks and discomfort involved which could include:

(a) dizziness and/fainting;

(b) haematoma formation during the pumped blood return;

(c) citrate toxicity, related to the rate and volume of citrated blood returned;

(d) blood loss if the procedure has to be terminated and it is considered unsafe to return donor blood remaining in the cell separator;

(e) chilling sensations on reinfusion;

(f) reactions to starch solutions used in white cell donation procedures.

4 General information with regard to the recipient's need for the donated product and the anticipated benefits.

5 Explain that as a voluntary donor, consent can be withdrawn at any stage of the procedure or of the apheresis programme.

6 Donor compensation. Health Authorities will consider sympathetically and decide promptly any claim on a donor for compensation for any injury or loss attributed to having donated a blood product by means of a cell separator.

Medical examination of donors

It is preferable to have an initial independent assessment of the health status of the donor by consulting the donor's general practitioner. Further medical examination should be carried out by the medical officer who undertakes the consent, to ensure that the donor meets the required standard of health. Temperature, pulse rate and blood pressure observations should be recorded on the operator's worksheet.

If there is clinical suspicion of cardiorespiratory disease (as indicated by the patient's history and the clinical examination) a specialist opinion should be sought.

Blood tests

The following blood tests *must* be included as a predonation screen:

blood grouping (ABO and Rh)

HB_sAg, HIV, TPHA

haemoglobin, white cell and platelet count

These additional tests *may* be indicated:

HLA typing

CMV antibody
total plasma proteins and immunoglobulins
liver function tests
urea and electrolytes
coagulation screen
screen for high titre anti A/B (for Group O platelet donors).

The results should be within the normal range for the age and sex of the donor.

Predonation white cell counts should exceed 4×10^9/litre and predonation platelet counts should exceed 150×10^9/litre.

Before white cell transfusions, a red cell cross-match, an HLA antibody screen or a lymphocytotoxic cross-match should normally be performed.

Frequency, volume and duration of the procedure

Donors should not normally be expected to donate more often than once a fortnight. The peak extracorporeal volume including the donation should not exceed 15% of the total blood volume. A donor should not normally donate platelets or white cells more often than twelve times a year. The volume of plasma removed should not exceed 600 ml (excluding the anticoagulant) without replacement plasma substitutes being used.

No more than 15 litres of plasma should be taken per annum and not more than 2.4 litres in any one month period or more than 1 litre per week. The duration of a machine donation procedure should not exceed 3 hours.

Donors who give the recommended maximum amount of plasma or cells annually should be given a full medical examination (including appropriate laboratory tests) once a year by an independent clinician.

Drugs and infusion fluids

It is recommended that the choice of drugs and other substances given to donors should be restricted and that normally only the following should be used, and then only with the consent of the donor.

Acid citrate dextrose
Heparin
Steroids
Dextran
Hydroxyethyl starch
Modified fluid gelatin
All albumin products

Records of cumulative doses of corticosteroids should be kept for each donor. When complications develop during the procedure, any other drugs (e.g.

protamine) may be used at the discretion of the consultant in charge of the cell separator, or his/her deputy.

Facilities

Accommodation

When cell separators are used for therapeutic purposes, a cardiac arrest team must be readily available. Ideally, cell separators should be operated in an area reserved exclusively for this work. This area should be adequate to allow a cardiac arrest team to operate. In addition, the area should provide working surfaces and washing facilities.

Resuscitation equipment

Full resuscitation facilities (as agreed by the hospital cardiac arrest team) must be available.

Staff

Training

Staff should be well trained and have regular instruction in resuscitation procedures and be familiar with the recommendations issued by the manufacturers of the cell separator in use. Written protocols should be available for each procedure undertaken and these should be strictly adhered to. The protocols should include a note of known complications of the procedure.

Normally, only doctors and qualified nurses should be trained to supervise the operation of cell separators. All members of staff operating the equipment must receive formal training either in their own or in another department. The consultant in charge must be responsible for arranging the training of staff.

The consultant in charge, in consultation with the nurse manager, must be satisfied that the necessary training has been completed before allowing staff to carry out procedures and should sign a statement to this effect. The employing Authority should be made aware that nurses operating cell separators are undertaking duties outside their normal province and should be provided with a list of these duties.*

The training should include consideration of the use and risks of anticoagulants and instruction in all aspects of the operation of the machine(s) in use.

* (HC(77)22) (Extended role of the nurse) (1979 (GEN) 46) for Scotland.

Training should also include consideration of the associated hazards and the action to be taken in the event of possible or actual harm to the patient.

Machine safety

Numerous types of cell separators are now available, but all operate on either a continuous or an intermittent flow principle usually involving a two arm venepuncture procedure allowing rapid return of citrated blood.

These systems consist of an instrumental device which will carry out whole blood separation, normally using a disposable apheresis set and a citrate and/or heparin anticoagulant solution. Such an integrated system withdraws blood from the donor, mixes it with anticoagulant in the required ratio, separates and collects the component selected, safely returning the remaining blood components to the donor/patient. For correct anticoagulant usage, refer to Appendix 2.

1 The machine should comply with the relevant aspects of the Health and Safety at Work Act.

2 The machine shall comply with the requirements of British Standard BS 5724: Part I: Safety of Medical Electrical Equipment. Before supply, the purchaser should obtain a completed MLQ1 and MLQ2 form from the manufacturer ensuring that the machine conforms with UK Health Department Guidance notes and should be purchased from a registered manufacturer.

3 When a new machine is being used on loan for assessment, the Health Authority should seek written assurances that the machine conforms to appropriate safety standards. The Department of Health has advised that health authorities should use the standard form of indemnity for equipment on loan, an example of which was issued to Health Authorities on 20 November 1986. A copy of the standard form is available from regional supplies departments. The intention of the form is that it should be used in any equipment loan transaction in which there is no payment made by the Authority in order to establish a contractual relationship and more effectively protect the Authority.

4 The supply of sterile, single use items and medical equipment should be purchased only from manufacturers who have been registered under the DHSS. 'Manufacturers Registration Scheme'. A list of currently approved manufacturers can be obtained from the regional supplies department. The machine should be correctly installed and commissioned in accordance with the manufacturer's recommendations.

5 If cell separators are in use which are fitted with reusable separation devices, strict sterilization procedures should be followed in accordance with the original *Code of Practice for the Clinical Use of Blood Cell Separators* (DHSS 1977).

Recommended safety features

HARNESS SOFTWARE

All tubing, separation bowls, collars, membranes and filters should preferably be single-use disposable items. When possible, they should normally be preconnected to ensure a sterile fluid pathway once venous access is achieved.

MANUAL OVERRIDE SYSTEM

A manual override system is essential to enable the operator to override any automated procedure at any stage to allow intervention in the event of complications occurring.

BLOOD FLOW MONITOR

Pressure sensors are required:

1 to monitor blood flow during withdrawal;

2 to monitor venous pressure during reinfusion.

If either of these situations occurs, a visual and audible alarm system should operate.

ANTICOAGULANT FLOW INDICATOR

A means of monitoring the rate of delivery of the anticoagulant throughout the procedure is essential.

BLOOD FILTER

The harness should incorporate blood filters to prevent aggregates formed during the procedure from entering the separator or from being returned to the patient/donor.

AIR-IN-LINE DETECTOR

The machine should include a protection system to ensure air infusion to the patient/donor cannot occur. The system should also incorporate a method of diverting accumulation of air from the patient reinfusion line should this occur due to technical problems.

The air detector must

activate an audible and visual alarm

activate line clamps to prevent further reinfusion
stop blood withdrawal and anticoagulant pumps

OPERATIVE PRESSURE MONITORS

Plasma filtration machines must be provided with a monitoring device to record the transmembrane pressure and a protective system to ensure that the machine will only operate between recommended preset ranges.

If the transmembrane pressure falls outside the preset ranges, an audible and visual alarm system should operate.

FLUID BALANCE

If systems incorporate automatic fluid balance control to ensure balance between collected components and replacement fluids, there should be a visual display, to allow the operator to monitor:

volume processed
cell/plasma removal rate
volume removed
volume reinfused

PROCEDURE PROGRAMMES

If a machine has more than one procedural programme available, there should be a visual display of the programme selected during the 'run' mode.

AUTOMATIC PRESSURE CUFF

If in use, there should be automatic inflation when the blood is being withdrawn and automatic deflation when blood withdrawal is stopped or during reinfusion if a single arm technique is in use.

BLOOD WARMERS

Blood warmers should be operated in accordance with manufacturers' instructions and should incorporate a thermostatic control device which gives an audible alarm when a temperature deviation occurs.

MACHINE MAINTENANCE

Cell separator machines should be serviced in accordance with the manufacturer's instructions. A planned maintenance scheme should be followed.

If maintenance, repairs and modifications are undertaken by a hospital department, this should be done in accordance with the procedures outlined in *Health equipment information*, HEI 98; *Management of equipment*, DHSS EU 26; and *Electric medical equipment guidance on documentation required for maintenance.* Cell separator machines should be cleaned after each procedure with a suitable decontaminating agent and a standard procedure for dealing with blood spillage should be adhered to.*

In the event of a mechanical failure of the machine, a service engineer should be contactable by telephone during normal working hours.

POWER FAILURE

To ensure donor/patient safety, the machine should automatically enter a standby mode once power returns after a temporary power failure. Also, a manual system for returning any remaining blood components to the patient/donor is desirable, particularly if the extra-corporeal volume is in excess of 200 ml and the power failure continues.

Appendix 1: Potential complications of therapeutic cell separator procedures

Mortality in therapeutic haemapheresis is estimated at 3 per 10 000 procedures.
Major hazards are related to

1 anticoagulants: citrate, heparin
2 type of replacement fluid
3 fluid and electrolyte balance
4 vascular access
5 haemolysis
6 air embolus
7 infection
8 paediatric usage

ANTICOAGULANTS

Citrate toxicity

This has been recorded in up to 15% of procedures and can lead to cardiac arrhythmias and death. It is related to the concentration of citrate anticoagulant used, the concentration of citrate in the replacement fluid, the rate of citrate infusion and to patient susceptibility. Citrate acts by chelating calcium ions and symptoms are due to

* The Howie Report: DHSS Code of Practice for the prevention of infection in clinical laboratories.

hypocalcaemia which are as follows; circumoral paraesthesiae, muscle twitching, nausea and/or vomiting, chills, syncope and tetany (rare).

NB Severe hypocalcaemia can occur without any of the above warning symptoms.

Avoidance

1 Use the manufacturer's recommended anticoagulant at the correct ratio.
2 If different citrate formulations are to be used, it is essential to monitor the citrate levels in the return line to the patient/donor and to monitor ionized calcium levels in the patient/donor to ensure the maximum citrate dose rate is not exceeded.
3 If patient susceptibility is suspected, for example impaired liver function, reinfuse at a slow rate and monitor for signs of hypocalcaemia.

NB It is safer to correct by stopping or slowing the reinfusion rate than to infuse concentrated calcium solutions—hypercalcaemia induced in this way can be as dangerous as hypocalcaemia.

Inadequate citration

If inadequate levels of citrate are achieved, this could lead to clotting in the extracorporeal cell separator circuit. This could either lead to the reinfusion of material with procoagulant activity and potentially precipitate disseminated intravascular coagulation (DIC), or cause haemolysis in the cell separator leading to reinfusion of haemolysed blood.

Avoidance

1 Use the manufacturer's recommended anticoagulant at the correct ratio.
2 Monitor the anticoagulant pump, the rate of delivery via the drip chamber and the volume of anticoagulant used throughout the procedure to ensure constant correct delivery of anticoagulant.
3 Monitor the separation chamber or the return line filter for evidence of clotting.
4 Monitor the colour of the separated plasma for evidence of haemolysis.

Adverse reactions to heparin

These include bleeding, allergy/anaphylaxis, dyspnoea and abdominal pain.

NB If Protamine is used to reverse heparin, the following adverse reactions can occur; chills and lightheadedness, allergy and/or anaphylaxis, dyspnoea and/or chest pain, and flushing.

Because of these adverse reactions and the prolonged effect of heparin, citrate is recommended as the anticoagulant of choice for most cell separator procedures and the use of heparin in normal donors should be avoided.

REPLACEMENT FLUIDS

The following materials have been used alone or in combination for fluid replacement in therapeutic exchange procedures:

plasma protein fraction (PPF)

human albumin solution 4.5% (HAS)
fresh frozen plasma (FFP)
whole blood and/or packed cells
volume expanders, e.g. modified fluid gelatin (MFG), Hydroxyethyl starch (HES), Haemaccel, Dextran; Crystalloids, e.g. Saline, Hartmans, etc.

No therapeutic materials should be added to HAS, blood or other blood products.

For plasma exchange procedures the choice of replacement fluid depends on the frequency and volume of the exchange procedure and the underlying disorder. However, in all patients it is important to maintain adequate levels of protein during the procedure as inadequate protein replacement can rapidly lead to hypovolaemia and hypotension.

Total replacement with albumin-containing solutions avoids this problem. Note that the maximum rate of removal should not exceed 20 ml/minute. Procedures can be done safely with a mixture of 50% crystalloid + 50% albumin *but* if frequency of exchange is more than once a week, the volume of the exchange is 1.5 × plasma volume, and replacement fluid is part crystalloid part albumin, albumin levels as well as other plasma proteins progressively fall. If replacement fluid is PPF or HAS only, albumin levels will be maintained, but there will be a progressive fall in levels of (i) coagulation factors (including fibrinogen and antithrombin III), (ii) immunoglobulins, (iii) complement and (iv) cholinesterase.

Reduction in coagulation factors can lead to bleeding episodes, particularly if there is a potential bleeding point, for example recent renal biopsy. This will be enhanced if heparin is used as the anticoagulant.

Reduction in anti-thrombin III levels (i) may predispose to thrombo-embolic episodes post exchange, (ii) reduces the effectiveness of heparin anticoagulation.

Reduction in cholinesterase levels can lead to prolonged periods of apnoea in response to the muscle relaxant suxamethonium used in general anaesthesia.

If volume expanders are used as part replacement, certain problems should be recognized.

1 Fluid overload precipitating congestive cardiac failure in the susceptible patient.
2 Allergic reactions particularly with dextrans.
3 Haemaccel has a high concentration of calcium which should *not* be mixed with citrated blood as this could produce clotting in the reinfusion blood line.

Complications of FFP

Allergy—can occur in up to 30% of cases
Anaphylaxis/pulmonary oedema—can be fatal (strong association with the use of FFP replacement and the fatalities attributed to plasma exchange)
Citrate toxicity—the combination of citrated plasma and citrated red cells can lead to severe citrate toxicity if rapid reinfusion rates used
ABO incompatibility—if mismatched plasma used
Respiratory distress syndrome—plasma contains HLA and/or neutrophil specific antibodies reactive with patient's leucocytes
Hepatitis
AIDS

NB Similar complications can occur if blood is used as part of the replacement fluid.

Avoidance

1 Only use FFP if essential. Currently, the only situation where FFP is the replacement fluid of choice is thrombotic thrombocytopenic purpura.
2 Use PPF or albumin as the major replacement fluid. Although occasional hypotensive or idiosyncratic reactions can occur to albumin preparations, they are much less common. It should be remembered that if the infusion rate exceeds 10 ml/minute, reactions are more likely to occur.
3 Single donor FFP units can be used at the end of an exchange procedure to maintain coagulation factors, immunoglobulin levels and cholinesterase levels if thought to be necessary.
4 Use of a 20 μ microaggregate filter reduces the incidence of allergic reactions. Microaggregates present in frozen/thawed plasma are probably responsible for the majority of allergic/anaphylactic reactions.
5 Ensure the patient is not IgA deficient. IgA deficient individuals usually possess anti-IgA and anaphylaxis is likely to occur in response to transfusion of any blood product containing IgA.

FLUID AND ELECTROLYTE BALANCE PROBLEMS

Hypervolaemia

Common in renal failure patients. Control is obtained by decreasing the volume of the replacement fluids, maintaining the albumin level, monitoring the BP and finishing the exchange in negative balance.

Hypovolaemia

Common in paediatric cases and small patients where the extracorporeal volume exceeds 10% of the patient's total blood volume. The initial signs are irritability, restlessness, yawning, drowsiness, cramps. Late signs are abdominal pain, vomiting, collapse.

Avoidance

1 Monitor BP.
2 Maintain albumin levels.
3 Increase reinfusion rate if signs of hypovolaemia occur.

Hyperviscosity states

Patients with hyperviscosity are usually hypervolaemic. If this type of patient is made hypovolaemic with an increase in the haematocrit before a reduction in the plasmaviscosity has been achieved, a hyperviscosity crisis can be precipitated, i.e. do not raise the patient's Hb/HCT until at least half the plasma volume has been exchanged during the first exchange procedure.

Electrolyte imbalance

Problems that can occur include hypokalaemia, hyponatraemia, hypocalcaemia, hypomagnesia and aluminium toxicity (high levels of aluminium present in some PPF and HAS preparations).

Avoidance

Choice of replacement fluid must be tailored to individual patient requirements which must be assessed prior to commencing the exchange procedure. PPF and HAS have normal sodium levels, but low levels of ionized calcium potassium and magnesium. Hence it may be necessary to normalize these levels by the addition of calcium and potassium to the replacement fluid.

In renal failure patients, it may be advantageous to omit potassium in the replacement fluid. Patients on diuretics or steroids may be more prone to potassium depletion and may require supplements in the replacement fluid.

NB Combination of hypocalcaemia and hypokalaemia can increase the likelihood of cardiac arrhythmias.

Chilling

Rapid reinfusion without using a blood warmer can cause 'chilling' and rigors. Patients suffering from sickle cell disease are prone to haemolysis and a blood warmer should be used.

NB In paraproteinaemias, cold haemagglutinin disease and cryoglobulinaemias, the cryocomponent may be active at relatively high temperatures and gelling or agglutination may occur in the extracorporeal circuit unless precautions are taken.

1 Check for presence of a cryocomponent in all paraproteinaemias referred for plasma exchange.

2 Assess the thermal amplitude of the cryocomponent if possible.

3 Ensure the temperature of the cell separator circuit does not fall below the critical level by using blood warmers to:

warm the prime solutions
warm the replacement fluid
warm the reinfused blood

4 Increase the temperature of the working environment.

COMPLICATIONS OF VASCULAR ACCESS

The safest venous access is by repeated use of the antecubital fossa veins. Where this is not possible, various types of vascular access have been used, none of which are without complications. Subclavian line/superior vena-caval catheters have led to vessel perforation, haemothorax, pneumothorax and infection and thrombosis. Femoral vein catheters have led to haemorrhage, thrombosis and infection.

Arterio-venous shunts have led to shunt site infections, which have been associated with recrudescence of the disease. Arterio-venous fistulae have led to gangrene and subsequent limb amputation, thrombosis and a CVA.

HAEMOLYSIS

Forcing blood by pump through a narrow orifice particularly when blood is concentrated to a high haematocrit, may result in haemolysis.

Avoidance

1 All the software must be carefully examined prior to setting up the machine to ensure there are no kinks or twists in the tubing.
2 Constant observation of the colour of the plasma to detect for the presence of haemolysis.
3 When using filtration machines, constant monitoring of the transmembrane pressure is essential and particular care taken if frequent episodes of low flow occur, as in this situation haemolysis is more likely to occur.

NB If haemolysis is suspected the procedure must be terminated as the return of damaged red cells to the patient/donor could precipitate DIC and mimic a haemolytic transfusion reaction.

AIR EMBOLUS

Most cell separators incorporate air detector devices in the reinfusion line. However, with the use of blood warmers and other software beyond the machine air detectors, there is a risk of air embolism if all the lines are not fully primed.

NB Never rely totally on 'fail/safe' alarm systems. Occasionally they can fail and constant monitoring of all reinfusion lines is necessary to prevent air embolism from occurring.

INFECTION

Equipment contamination

Do not leave a machine primed for longer than 1 hour prior to its use.

Bacterial infection

If bacterial contamination has occurred during the set-up and priming procedure, there is a risk of causing a severe bacteraemia, which could be fatal in an immunosuppressed patient. Plasma exchange depletes immunoglobulin if PPF or albumin is used as the replacement fluid. The combination of low immunoglobulins and immunosuppressive therapy predisposes the patient to infection. Prophylactic administration of immune serum globulin in patients particularly at risk should only be considered under special circumstances.

Viral infection

If FFP is used as the replacement fluid, hepatitis, particularly the non-A non-B variety is a potential risk and can be lethal. FFP should only be used for TTP or when specific replacement of plasma deficient factors is required.

PAEDIATRIC USAGE

Protocols necessary for plasma exchange in children (from the Hospital for Sick Children, Great Ormond Street)

1 Record child's dry weight and resting BP.
2 Cross-match and prime machine with whole blood for the first exchange and subsequent exchanges if the pre Hb is < 9 g/dl.
3 For children < 30 kg, prime through to the return line with blood and/or plasma. If < 20 kg, always prime with whole blood.
4 PPF used as replacement fluid 80–120 ml/kg.
5 Use FFP with a 20 μ microaggregate filter at end of exchange from third day to replace depleted clotting factors.
6 Use a blood warmer on the return line.
7 Worse aspect to the child is insertion of lines. Great Ormond Street Hospital have found A-V shunts to be the most successful and least traumatic to the child.

NB If possible, use a cell separator that has a small extracorporeal volume. Most continuous flow filtration (membrane) machines are suitable, but the disadvantage is that they require relatively high flow rates and usually require an invasive form of vascular access.

Contraindications to plasma exchange in children

1 Heart failure.
2 Uncontrollable hypertension.
3 Renal biopsy/major surgery 5 days before plasma exchange.

Appendix 2: Guidelines for operators outlining standards of care for patients and donors undergoing blood cell separation

A consultant fully experienced in the operation of cell separators has overall responsibility for the health and welfare of patients/donors and for the observance of the codes of practice. Registered general nurses are responsible for nursing care aspects.

To provide optimal care, procedures should be carried out by a team of two personnel, one of whom should be a specifically trained registered nurse. The person who prepares the machine, ideally the registered nurse, will have the responsibility for its operation.

The nurse in charge has responsibility for:
the physical and psychological needs of the patient/donor
making sure that support facilities are available and functioning
completing a comprehensive record/work sheet

making sure there is instruction on post-procedural care and subsequent follow-up of patient/donor.

Standards and monitoring required to prevent complications

The clinical hazards associated with procedures and the avoidance of such complications are clearly outlined in Appendix 1.

In order to minimize operational error, the following should apply.

1 Information required with reference to specific patient/donor management.

(a) The physical and psychological condition of the patient/donor.

(b) Any associated nursing care required.

(c) The basic parameters required to establish the total blood and plasma volume: height, weight and Hct (relevant to the volume to be removed or exchanged and the anticoagulant ratio to be used).

(d) The details of current drug therapy, particularly anticonvulsants, anti-arrhythmics and steroids. It may be necessary to modify drug regimens or to give supplemental doses in order to maintain the desired drug concentration in the blood, especially when large quantities of plasma are to be removed.

(e) If there is a history of cardiac valvular disease, specialist advice about antibiotic prophylaxis should be sought.

2 A written protocol for each procedure which must be specific for the machine in use must be available. It should include a detailed description of the entire procedure.

3 Maintenance of records and care plans, which include details of the following:

(a) patient identification and diagnosis
(b) the responsible medical officer and operator's signature
(c) type of procedure and serial number of machine
(d) batch number of solutions and software
(e) method of access
(f) volume and rate of blood processed
(g) nature and volume of anticoagulant and replacement fluids
(h) duration of the procedure
(i) details of any medication given
(j) adverse reactions and their treatment.

4 All nurses/operators must be aware of and be able to recognize the complications which may arise during the procedure and be fully conversant with the corrective or preventive action to be taken.

5 If the nurse/operator considers operating conditions unsafe or he/she does not feel competent to undertake the procedure, he/she should not proceed before seeking advice from the consultant in charge of the unit.

6 Results of appropriate laboratory tests itemized in the protocol for the procedure concerned should be available so that advice concerning the intervention or adjustment to treatment can be sought.

7 It is the nurse/operator's responsibility to ensure that the operating standards for the management of complications are complied with when undertaking procedures on patients or donors. These should include details of the following:

(a) procedure in the event of a respiratory or cardiac arrest and application of the techniques involved and the equipment in use

(b) procedure following accident or incident

(c) action in the event of fire or bomb alert.

8 Any drug, anticoagulant or IV solution given to a patient/donor should be checked before administration, or introduction into the machine. This checking must be carried out by two people, one of whom must be a qualified Medical Officer or a Registered General Nurse. For example:

(a) the appropriate method of anticoagulation must comply with prescribed policy for the particular procedure

(b) the consultant responsible for cell separators or his/her deputy shall prescribe the replacement regimen required for a particular procedure or patient treatment

(c) the general guidelines for infusion or transfusion are known and applied.

Technical aspects of the procedure

HARNESSING AND PRIMING OF THE MACHINE

1 Check that all disposable equipment, solutions and sterile packages available are in date, undamaged and that batch/lot numbers are recorded.

2 Recheck for harness faults during installation, priming and running of the machine.

3 The batch numbers of faulty harnesses should be reported to the manufacturer, so that the batch can be investigated and withdrawn if necessary.

4 Use aseptic technique when connecting tubing and solutions.

5 Check that all alarm systems are functioning.

The above checks will assist in the prevention of the following:

bacterial infection caused by contamination during setting-up and priming

mechanical haemolysis caused by twisted or trapped tubes

the entry of air into the circuit caused by increased pressure in the extracorporeal circuit or loose connections.

THE DETECTION OF FAULTS IN THE AUTOMATIC PROGRAMMING

Check that operation of the machine is correct for the given programme and that the programme is maintained throughout the procedure. The displayed function should be recorded at regular intervals.

MANUAL OVERRIDE

Manual override in automatic systems is necessary in the following circumstances:

Citrate toxicity

stop or slow down reinfusion until symptoms subside.

Hypovolaemia

stop withdrawal of blood and commence reinfusion until the patient/donor's condition is stable.

Major complications

terminate the procedure without returning any machine contents.

Examples of major complications:
- Haemolysis
- Under anticoagulation
- Severe complications of vascular access
- Allergic reactions
- Haemorrhage
- Disease related 'crisis' (e.g., myasthenic crisis)
- Cardiac/respiratory arrest
- Serious faults in the equipment.

Minor complications include:
- Venospasm or vasovagal reaction
  slow down or stop the procedure until the patient recovers
- Haematoma
  apply pressure and resite the needle
- Hypothermia
  slow down or stop the procedure and check the function of blood warmer. Take appropriate measures to warm the patient/donor.

VENOUS FLOW

1 Visually check that venous and anticoagulant flow rates are appropriate.
2 Ensure satisfactory maintenance of the pressure cuff, if in use.
3 Check for gelling or agglutination.

REINFUSION CIRCUIT

1 Check that no clotted or haemolysed blood or air emboli are delivered to the patient/donor.
2 Ensure that an adequate reinfusion rate is maintained.

SEPARATION EXIT

1 Ensure that the appropriate undamaged blood components are removed at the required rate.
2 According to the machine in use, check that transmembrane pressure is maintained or that no excessive vibration or overheating occurs.
3 Observe for leaks in separator.

PUMP FUNCTION

1 Adjust the pump speeds as necessary to ensure smooth and efficient operation.
2 Check for any tubing occlusion, particularly in the pump heads.

MAINTENANCE OF FLUID BALANCE

1 Exclude deviation from machine readouts by measuring input and output of fluids.
2 Monitor reinfusion and draw flow rates.

Completion of procedure

On completion of the procedure, the patient/donor should be given appropriate post-procedural advice and care.

Provision for disposal of waste and used disposable equipment should be made in accordance with the Health and Safety Commission Report 1982 *The Safe Disposal of Clinical Waste* (ISBN 0-11-883641-2).

Cell separator machines should be cleaned after each procedure with a suitable decontaminating agent. 'The Howie Report', DHSS *Code of Practice for the Prevention of Infection in Clinical Laboratories* should be followed. Staff should take care to protect themselves when using cleaning agents and solutions by wearing appropriate clothing including masks and gloves.

Appendix 3: Donor consent form (cell separators)

1 I .... (*Full name*)

of .... (*Full address*)

hereby acknowledge that I have volunteered to donate blood by means of a cell separator. The nature and purpose of the donation of blood by those means and the risks involved to the donor have been explained to me by:

Dr. .... *

I hereby consent to the donation of

by means of a cell separator and I agree to undergo medical assessment which will also involve giving a sample of my blood for tests including HIV. I consent to such further or alternative operative measures or treatment as may be found necessary during the course of the donation.

Signature of volunteer donor ....

Date ....

2 I confirm that I have explained the nature and purpose of this procedure to the person who signed the above form of consent.

Signature of doctor ....

Date ....

* The explanation must be given by a medical practitioner.

Appendix

Standards and reference preparations—blood products and related substances (National Institute for Biological Standards and Control).

Material	Code No.	Units/ampoule	Description
Factor VIII: C concentrate	80/556	3.9 IU	3rd IS
Factor VIII-related activities in plasma:			
Factor VIII:C		0.60 IU	
Factor VIII:Ag	87/718	0.91 IU	2nd IS
vWF:RCoF		0.84 IU	
vWF:Ag		0.91 IU	
Factor VIII:C Plasma	88/584	0.67 IU	16th BS
Blood coagulation factors Plasma:			
VIII:Ag		0.85	
vWF:RCof	87/658	0.71	3rd BS
vWF:Ag		0.81	
Factor IX		0.81	
AT III		0.88	
Protein C		0.91	
Factor VIII:C concentrate	88/590	3.9 IU	8th BS
Factor VIII concentrate, porcine	86/514	9.1 U	1st BS
Factor II, IX, X concentrate	84/681	II: 10.8 IU IX: 10.7 IU X: 9.8 IU	1st IS
Factor II, VII, IX, X plasma	84/665	II: 0.83 IU VII: 0.91 IU IX: 0.80 IU X: 0.81 IU	1st IS
Factor IX concentrate	87/532	II: 7.1 IU IX: 6.3 IU X: 6.1 IU	2nd BWS
Factor VIII reagents:			
Phospholipid, bovine brain	86/516	10 mg/ml	NIBSC
Bovine Factor V	88/614	–	NIBSC
Human serum	85/500	–	NIBSC

Material	Code No.		Units/ampoule	Description
Thrombin, human	70/157		100 IU	1st IS
Plasmin	77/588		10 IU	2nd IRP
Plasminogen (glu-)	78/646		10 U	1st BS
Streptokinase–streptodornase	62/7		3100 IU	1st IS
t-PA (tissue plasminogen activator)	86/670		850 IU	2nd IS
Urokinase	66/46		4800 IU	IRP
Ancrod	74/581		55 IU	1st IRP
Batroxobin (moojeni)	75/527		65 U	1st BS
Heparin, porcine mucosal	82/502		1780 IU	4th IS
Heparin, low molecular weight	85/600	Anti-Xa thrombin inhibition	1680 IU 665 IU	1st IS
Protamine	54/5		–	1st IRP
Factor Xa, bovine	75/595		1 U	NIBSC reagent
Antithrombin III, plasma	72/1		0.9 IU	1st IRP
Prekallikrein activator (PKA), human	79/572		78.9 units/ml	1st BS
Prekallikrein activator (PKA), human	82/530		85 IU	1st IS
Beta thromboglobulin (Beta-TG), human	83/501		500 IU	1st IS
Platelet factor 4 (PF_4), human	83/505		400 IU	1st IS
Protein C, plasma	86/622		0.82 IU	1st IS
Ferritin, human liver	80/602		9.7 μg	1st IS
Ferritin, human spleen for immunoassay	80/578		9.7 μg	–
Anti-D immunoglobulin, human	68/419		300 IU	1st IRP
Anti-D (Rho) antibodies human	72/229		11.5 IU	1st BS
Human serum vitamin B_{12}	81/563		320 pg	1st BS
Human C-reactive protein	85/506		0.049 IU	1st IS

IS = International Standard, IRP = International Reference Preparation,
BS = British Standard, BWS = British Working Standard,
NIBSC = NIBSC Reagent.

All these materials are available from: Division of Haematology, National Institute for Biological Standards and Control, Blanche Lane, South Mimms, Potters Bar, Herts EN6 3QG, UK.

Index

Page numbers in **bold** indicate tables and those in *italic* indicate figures.